1980

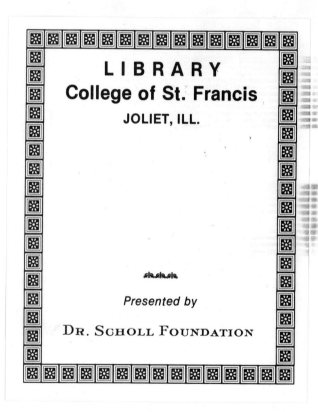

Social Policies and Programs on Aging

Social Policies and Programs on Aging

What Is and What Should Be
in the Later Years

Louis Lowy
Boston University

LexingtonBooks
D.C. Heath and Company
Lexington, Massachusetts
Toronto

Library of Congress Cataloging in Publication Data

Lowy, Louis.
  Social policies and programs on aging.

  Includes bibliographies and index.
  1. Aged—Governmental policy—United States. 2. Aged—United States.
3. United States—Social policy. I. Title.
HQ1064.U5L69   362.6'0973   78-55355
ISBN 0-669-02342-6

Published simultaneously in Canada

Printed in the United States of America

International Standard Book Number: 0-669-02342-6

Library of Congress Catalog Card Number: 78-55355

To the aspirations, efforts, and
accomplishments of the members of the
Boston University Gerontology Center
in the service of our older
population everywhere

Contents

Contents

List of Figures
and Tables

Preface

A few years ago, while working on the manuscript for my book, *Social Work with the Aging: The Challenge and Promise of the Later Years*, I planned a companion volume that would focus on the social policies and programs affecting the aging. As a practitioner in the field of aging I became aware very early that "policy enacts practice" and that "practice enacts policy." Alfred Kahn's dictum was literally translated for me in my social work activities on the direct-service level as well as on the levels of planning, policy shaping and policy implementation through administration and management of social service programs. The complementarity of policy and practice is evident in all spheres of our endeavors, but too often we are blind to this evidence when we get immersed in one or the other aspect of our work. Every so often the blinding veil has to be lifted, and we have to become conscious of the interrelationships and connections between policy and practice.

As a teacher and educator I have tried to convey Kahn's dictum and demonstrate its all-pervasive truth to my students here and abroad. At times I have succeeded in my efforts; at others I have not. (One might say, this is a truism of the lot of every teacher.) Hopefully I have succeeded more frequently than I have failed. Fortunately there is some evidence that a sizable number of my students have incorporated this dictum in their practice as they perform their daily tasks of providing services to older people in many settings, such as long-term-care facilities, home-care programs, state offices on aging, counseling agencies, hospitals, mental health clinics, multiservice centers, legal research and protective service programs, advocacy groups, federal departments, international bodies, institutions of higher learning, adult education programs, gerontology centers, and many more. And it makes no difference where, when, and from whom these students learned to integrate policy with practice (and vice versa), as long as they do it and do it well, informed by competence and compassion.

This book attempts to provide an overview of some of our present social policies and programs as they relate to older people in our society. Since these policies and programs are of major import to the human-service practitioner, it also defines issues and options and makes recommendations for change—what is now and also what should be.

An increasing wave of publications in the field of gerontology offsets the meager diet of the gerontological literature of the not-so-recent past. This is all to the good, although there are bound to be duplications, overlaps, and repetitions. At the same time, many of these publications add new dimensions, new viewpoints, and new conceptual frameworks to a field that has been neglected far too long. These developments are exciting as we experience the advent of new ideas that are likely to have considerable impact not only on the aging population but on all age groups. Although this book draws heavily, and appropriately, on the extant information and knowledge base in the area of policies and programs, it is geared first and foremost to the human-service practitioner, that is, the social worker, nurse, physician, mental health specialist, occupational therapist, counselor, clergyman, planner, administrator, teacher, and educator. It is also written for those who are part of the informal service network, as family members, neighbors, and friends of older persons are nowadays referred to in the language of "bureaucrateeze."

It is impossible to list all people who directly and indirectly had a share in the efforts, thoughts, and ideas that went into the preparation of this book. Nevertheless special thanks are due to Ellen Parker, who assisted greatly in the review of the literature and in pulling together disparate materials. Her enthusiasm, interest, level of competence, and understanding of the subject proved exemplary. Doreen Bender and Gail Sendecke deserve special commendation for their patience in deciphering my handwritten sheaves of paper and coming up with the typed manuscript in the nick of time.

Last but not least, let me express special gratitude to my practitioner colleagues in the field, to my faculty colleagues in the Boston University School of Social Work and at the Boston University Gerontology Center, and to my former and present students here and abroad who have taught me much and stimulated me in my pursuits as a gerontological social worker and teacher.

At a time of increasing perplexity, of changing value orientations, of economic uncertainties and demographic shifts, of political upheavals and a questioning of traditional beliefs and assumed certainties, we need to examine our present social policies vis-à-vis all age groups, not just those affecting the aging, as to their impact on people's lives, and to be sensitive to the unintended consequences of well-meaning intentions. We should also examine how our present and future policies and programs are likely to affect the quality of life of everybody—young and old—and how we can participate in shaping policies that answer to the values of a humane, compassionate, caring, and socially just society.

Acknowledgments

Acknowledgments are made to the members of the Professional Advisory Committee of the Massachusetts Department of Elder Affairs (DEA), who have stimulated many ideas and thoughts for this book and who have contributed many proposals related to social-policy issues and questions affecting older people throughout the country; to James Callahan, Jr., former secretary of Elder Affairs of the Commonwealth—now director of the Levinson Policy Institute at Brandeis University—and to members of his staff at DEA, notably Richard Le Blanc and John Peterson, Steve Day and Ann Downing, who have offered many ideas and have made many suggestions toward shaping policy and programs on aging in Massachusetts and other parts of the United States. Special acknowledgments are made to Legal Research and Services for the Elderly in Washington, D.C., for their various compilations of programmatic information, particularly in the areas of social security, medicare, and medicaid, that have been most valuable and useful to me and to my students. A number of my colleagues have made critical comments and have offered useful advice; all these contributions have found their way into the final document.

Acknowledgments

Social Policies
and Programs
on Aging

1 Introduction

This book is intended primarily for practitioners in the field of aging and for those students in colleges and universities who are preparing for such practice. They are expected to become familiar with the context of our social policies on aging, with existing gerontological programs, services, and benefits for older persons that are the result either of deliberate social policies or of ad hoc improvisations that may become social policies.

Practitioners, be they social workers, nurses, allied health professionals, or social planners, by their actions are not merely implementing such social policies, they are, in fact, enacting social policies themselves. This awareness is of crucial importance to the conduct of every practitioner's behavior. The practitioner directly involved in the provision of services to clients can play an important role in the formulation of and is instrumental to the execution of the policies that guide service organizations. In practice the separation of policy formulation from execution is a delicate division; aware and experienced practitioners often exercise considerable discretion in executing broad directives and thus shape as well as discharge the requirements of organizational policies.[1]

Our older population whether individuals, members of families, groups, or organizations, or citizens in their neighborhoods—is the ultimate beneficiary or victim of social policies, regardless of how they are enacted. For this reason every practitioner in the field of aging must be aware of the assumptions on which such policies rest, what the major social programs affecting the lives of older people are, and what issues need to be addressed now and in the future to effect a more equitable share for our growing older population.

This book affirms the conception of social justice as formulated by Rawls as a rationale for an equitable social policy for the aging in our society.[2] Rawls proposes that differences in life prospects are just if the greater expectations of the more advantaged improve the expectations of the least advantaged and that the basic structure of society is just throughout provided that the advantages of the more fortunate further the well-being of the least fortunate. Society's structure is perfectly just provided that the prospects of the least fortunate are as great as they can be.

We are a long way from such a social structure. But the vision of a just society shall guide our efforts, no matter how stumbling and halting, on the rocky road toward achieving a better life not only for the old but also for the young and the middle-aged. Only an age-integrated society can succeed in creating a full life-experience for all its members that epitomizes the highest quality of human existence.

Organization of the Book

Based on the rationale of social justice this book takes as its central theme the concept of human needs interfaced with their particular manifestations among older people. *Needs* are defined here as human strivings to fulfill existential conditions that are basic to insure the survival of people as wholistic human beings, biological, psychological, social, cultural, and spiritual. That is why Maslow's formulation of a needs hierarchy is utilized. Maslow postulates that higher types of human needs can only be gratified after lower types have been gratified. Since only unmet needs become problems, the needs concept forestalls the identification of aging as problematic and older people with being ipso facto social problems. After delineating particular human-needs areas and sketching existing policies (most of them in the public arena), a description of present programs, services, and benefits follows, including an enumeration of major policy issues and options for change.

By choice this book is practical and selective. It concentrates on those need areas that are of major existential import; therefore no claim for inclusiveness is made. It is an outgrowth of my course "Social Policy and Programs on Aging" for graduate students of social work, nursing, and allied health professionals, given over the past ten years at Boston University. Major objectives of this course have been to sensitize and alert students to the byways and pathways of social policies on aging, to familiarize them with basic programs and services, to help them make the best possible use of existing programs for the benefit of their clients, patients, and constituents, to instill a critical attitude toward our social policies, and to stimulate them to design better policies through direct practice or through policy shaping in planning and administrative positions. The ultimate consumer of a social policy on aging is always the individual older person (and his or her family) whose well-being must be safeguarded, since even well-meaning and well-designed social policies may be harmful in their unintended consequences.

In chapter 2 of the book data on the "graying" of America are provided to present a demographic profile and selected characteristics of our aging population for present and future policy making.

Chapter 3 sketches the historical road from the first White House Conference in 1961 to the planning of the third conclave in 1981 in Washington. It delineates our societal context and the conditions that create deliberate or ad hoc social policy on aging, based on attitudes and values, information and knowledge, and configurations of power. It concludes with a description of two major legislative foundations—the Social Security Act as amended and the Older Americans Act as amended—that have led to the formation of an "aging network" during the 1970s.

In chapter 4 our major income policies and programs represented through the remarkable complexities of our social security system and pension plans, are discussed. Chapter 5 reviews health policies, health programs and services, including such major financing mechanisms as medicare and medicaid. Long-term care, nursing homes, the hospice movement, and mental health policies and issues are addressed. Chapter 6 deals with our housing policies, exemplified by our housing laws, and living-arrangement options that become increasingly available.

In chapter 7 the formidable array of formal social and support services are reviewed and related to the informal assistance network extant in many communities. The "service strategy" is in clear view here, in contrast to the "income strategy" treated in earlier chapters.

Chapter 8 elucidates the emergence and development of advocacy, the organization and involvement of the elderly population and their impact on the design, shaping, and implementation of social policy for older people and the rest of society.

The last chapter summarizes present trends and attempts to carve out policy and program directions for tomorrow's agenda.

Aging and Social Policy

The elderly population in the United States is growing at a faster rate than any other age group within the population. By the year 2030, two of every eleven Americans will be over 65 years of age. One of the astounding revolutionary phenomena of our times is that in the more affluent parts of the world, for the first time in history, *"le troisiéme âge"* (the third age) and, indeed already *le quatriéme âge* (the fourth age) have become a reality. Around 1900 the average life span for a person was 40 years of age. Today more white women and white men in the United States reach the age of 72 and 68, respectively, than ever before. There is still much to be done to enable those who have been discriminated against in our social structure to catch up. Some of those who live under "double jeopardy" (discriminated against because of age *and* race) are: blacks, Chicanos, American Indians, and Asian Americans. However, the very fact that we have arrived at all at a *troisiéme âge*, in the life cycle means that our social institutions have to be redesigned to include the middle and later years of life. The idea of preparing ourselves for only the first two ages of life has become obsolete. Aging is a worldwide phenomenon. As the world approaches the year 2000 there is a rising level of consciousness about old people everywhere. There are more of them, and they are becoming more visible. The decision by the United Nations to hold a World Assembly on Aging in 1982 reflects this concern.

We have learned a good deal about the biological, physiological, and psychological processes of aging, although we are still at the threshold of such knowledge; we have learned a good deal about the sociological, cultural, economic, and political aspects of aging, but we have barely crossed the threshold of this type of knowledge. Natural, behavioral and social scientists, health and social practitioners, planners and researchers, politicians and legislators have demonstrated their growing interest in aging and in the aging population and have joined in learning more about the processes of growing older since they frequently are forced to translate data and knowledge—incomplete as they may be—into action. The emergence of the Gerontological Society since 1945, with its four sections of the Biological Sciences, Clinical Medicine, the Behavioral and Social Sciences, and Planning, Practice and Research, illustrates both the diversity of multidisciplinary endeavors and the imperative of integrating this diversity into a more unitary discipline. That is why gerontology as a science of aging is still emerging and geriatrics as a medical specialty is still seeking recognition in its own right among medical practitioners and researchers.

Everywhere around us decisions are made about older people, although few are made by older people themselves. These decisions, however, not only affect the elderly, they also affect their older and younger children and grandchildren, their fellow citizens in all walks of life, and generations not yet born. They affect the structure and functions of social institutions, such as families and their life patterns, business, commerce and labor, agriculture and banking, the health care system, the legal and social services, housing and ecology, the gross national product, consumer spending, educational and cultural institutions, and indeed the life-style of millions of people.

Although some attitudes about growing old have remained the same regardless of when or where they were expressed, it is clear that images of aging in this country have changed during the past two centuries. The types of roles Americans expected elderly men and women to fulfill have varied considerably over time. As a result, different perceptions of old people have evolved.

Before the Civil War, the old were considered more venerable, because they provided essential services. A different perspective gradually, but increasingly, emerged. By the time of the Great Depression Americans were describing the aged as "problems" because they imagined the old to be sick, poor, and useless. Recently, there has been a slow but growing tendency to reevaluate our notions about the social value of old age. We are gradually beginning to appreciate and utilize the diverse potentials of our elderly citizens.

The graying of America will bring many changes—some of them already are perceptible. Politicians will feel increasing pressure from their elderly constituents for new social programs. The economy will have to carry a much bigger burden in pension and social security benefits. Business will alter the products it makes and the way it sells them.

Let me list here a few implications for an "aging America." If retirement restrictions are completely lifted, additional employment opportunities for older persons will have to be developed; for the elderly on relatively fixed incomes, solutions will have to be found to meet inflationary housing, medical, and living costs. Second careers may become more common, and the number of older women in the job market can be expected to increase; a shorter work week will provide more leisure time and, perhaps, will allow more people of all ages to hold jobs; recreational facilities will be built for older adults, not just for their children and grandchildren. Life-long learning will indeed become a reality, creating many more educational opportunities for older persons, with emphasis on innovative approaches to teaching. As the elderly become more aware of their own potential for influence they will become their own advocates for social, economic, and political reforms. More housing options for the elderly will be needed and created. An incresing number of day-care centers, day hospitals, and other community services will provide alternatives to nursing homes. Through cross-generational activities, young and old will discover potential richness and concerns of the elderly within the context of a different age stratification. In short, the lives of all, today and tomorrow, will be significantly touched and affected by the demographic revolution caused by the advent of the third and the fourth ages in the history of humankind.

What Is Social Policy?

Freeman and Sherwood offer four definitions of social policy. Social policy as a philosophical concept is the principle whereby members of large organizations and political entities collectively seek enduring solutions to the problems that affect them. Social policy as a product consists of the conclusions reached by persons concerned with the betterment of community conditions and social life and with the amelioration of deviance and social disorganization. Social policy as a process consists of actions by which organizations maintain an element of stability and at the same time seek to improve conditions for their members. Social policy as a framework for action is both product and process. It assumes the availability of a policy that is to be implemented within the context of potential changes in the values, structure, and conditions of the group affected.[3] It is the latter definition that will be used throughout this book, since we are concerned primarily with the results, that is, products, of such policies that in their implementation become translated into programs and/or services rather than with an analysis of the policy-making processes per se.

In an orderly world there are several basic tasks that are systematically undertaken by policy makers that should result in a policy. These tasks are: planning, program development, program implementation, and evaluation.

Planning includes the identification of goals, predicated on assumptions or knowledge about values and existing conditions of a situation to be changed toward that goal, for example, to assume an adequate income in retirement in accord with the prevailing American standard of living.

Program development refers to the design of specific interventive activities toward goal achievement. It is concerned with selecting a strategy that is likely to overcome barriers and resistances that impede the achievement of the desired goals. For example, a variety of plans or proposals that would assure such an income would be designed, taking into account costs and benefits to the elderly and nonelderly, sources of financing and funding, and impacts on the economy and on people's lives. At the same time the feasibility of congressional action in favor of such plans would be evaluated and strategic techniques developed to make adoption of a viable plan more likely.

Program implementation is the actual operation of the program design as finally promulgated in practice—the translation of the program plans into concrete action that affects the target population as well as peripheral and tangential groups. As an illustration one would cite the operation of the various income-maintenance mechanisms under the relevant titles of the Social Security Act designed for retired persons.

Evaluation provides the basis for the policy makers' decisions concerning the continuation, changes, expansion, or elimination of programs directed toward the goal as originally formulated and subsequently amended. In our example evaluation would review how these social security programs work, whether they deliver what was expected, what unanticipated consequences have resulted, and how they can be changed to take into account changing circumstances—for example, an increasing-age population, earlier retirements, shrinkage of available funds, political repercussions, and so on—and yet honor the promise of its original goal.

Admittedly this is a thumbnail sketch of a complex process that, in reality, is neither that orderly nor that systematically carried out. In addition, we do not live in a tidy, orderly world. In fact, many programs and services in the field of aging are more often the result of ad hoc measures, usually responding to crisis conditions, political pressures, and opportunities, economic exigencies such as the energy crisis in the 1970s and 1980s, and humanitarian motives. Thus the theme of the 1971 White House Conference on Aging, "Toward a National Policy on Aging," although laudable in intent, could not deliver in reality.

Our social policies toward the aging have moved toward selective assumption of societal responsibility and away from reliance on exclusive kin or filial responsibility, toward acceptance of rightful entitlement of benefits rather than dependency on charitable supports that are stigmatized, and toward more institutional services geared to meet individual requirements rather than residual, undifferentiated services. Despite this progress, the gap between need and action is wide, knowledge has been utilized inadequately, the elderly are still given low priority in allocation of funds and resources. Negative attitudes and stereotypes persist among the public as well as professionals, and no coherent, comprehensive social policy toward the aged has as yet been formulated in the United States, despite an attempt to do so during the 1971 White House Conference.

The social-welfare system in the United States has gradually evolved into a series of laws, benefits, programs, and services for older people that, presumably, respond to some of their needs and assist in coping with some of their developmental tasks. Social-welfare functions in relation to meeting needs and solving problems of older people can be divided into three parts: (1) the curative function, also termed a therapeutic, adjustmental function, provides for the solution of problems that have occurred as a result of malfunctioning within the individual or because of external factors; (2) the preventive function attempts to meet needs before they turn into problems, and consequently, human needs have to be identified well in advance; and (3) the promotional, enhancement-oriented function concerns itself with advancing the social standard for all older people by reducing many risk conditions that beset old age specifically, it thereby can lead to the achievement of the highest level of physical and social functioning of which persons are capable. This orientation is most in accord with a developmental rather than a residual view of social welfare.

In the immediate past, social welfare has been mostly concerned with alleviating existing problems and with helping in the adjustment of people to cope with conditions in their environment. Recently, there has been increasing recognition that efforts have to be expanded to insure that known risk conditions should be reduced as far as possible. The goal has been to get people to accept inevitable developmental phenomena of aging as normal tasks of living in later years and to minimize traumatic effects on this adjustmental process. In other words, people have to learn to consider "aging" as normal as "adolescence," recognizing that it has many biological, physiological, psychological, and sociological concomitants.

We still tend to look at the aging population as one beset with problems and to define it as a social problem rather than as a social group. Our youth-and work-oriented society, while ignoring, if not rejecting, the aged, has created situations that call for new approaches to meet the needs of its aging population. This is why a nonstigmatized network of health and social services is needed to reduce the vicissitudes of old age and to assist the aged to solve the normal problems of living that essentially are not of their making.[4]

Agenda for Social Policy on Aging

A series of social-goal statements identified by older persons and their organizations, by professionals working in the field, and by political leaders constitute the agenda of our social policy on aging that will certainly continue to surface during the 1981 White House Conference. These social goals include:

1. Assurance of an adequate income for every older person through a federally administered system of income security that is protected against inflation, devaluation of the dollar, and pension loss.
2. Reduction or abatement of federal, state, and local taxes for older persons and also a reduction of rates of public utilities such as transportation, telephone, gas, electricity, and so forth.
3. Reorganization and reordering of the physical and mental health delivery system with stress on case finding, early detection, treatment, rehabilitation, prevention, group practice, and home assistance; development of an all-inclusive prepaid national health-insurance system to remove financial worries and to assure cost control.
4. Provision of increased public social services divorced from financial needs.
5. Development of additional social and community services that would include many additional social services for older people and for research and demonstration projects leading to newer or improved programs to aid them.
6. Increase in older persons' housing options in urban and rural areas and eligibility of single persons for moderate-income and rental housing that is now available only to couples; in addition, automatic inclusion of a battery of social services in all public-housing projects designed for the elderly.
7. Inclusion in national service-programs opportunities for older people who are able and willing and in a position to provide services for people with problems in all age groups.
8. Expansion of the Manpower Development and Training Act and Area Development Act to help older workers and those in the middle years make the best possible use of training opportunities in communities and to prepare for second careers.
9. Provision of a pool for part-time employment opportunities for older people and preretirement counseling services sponsored under industry, management, and labor.

10. Increase in the federal contribution for the building of long-term-care facilities, provision of more uniform standards for nursing homes, and provision of more uniform quality standards for nursing-home care with enforcement possibilities. Removal of institutional stigma from institutions for the aged who are chronically ill.

11. Development of increased geriatric treatment facilities for the mentally ill and disabled and halfway houses for those who are released from hospitals and mental health institutions.

12. Provisions of a continuum of home health services and medical care services for the physically ill as well as the mentally ill in their own homes or homes of relatives.

13. Provision of an increased program of foster and boarding care for the elderly.

14. Development of day-care centers, recreation centers, and outreach programs for those who cannot take advantage of existing recreational facilities.

15. Increase in educational and cultural opportunities under adult education and cultural auspices.

16. Development of a more uniform program of accessible social services, particularly homemaker, health aides, protective, consumer information, legal assistance, friendly visitor, meals-on-wheels, and multiservice centers.

17. Creation of nutritional programs coupled with social, educational, and recreational services to improve the nutrition of older people and to assist in alleviating incipient personal problems.

18. Provision of improved transportation facilities to counteract physical isolation and to advance the mobility of older persons.

19. Development of short-range and long-range plans by all professions and organizations (governmental and nongovernmental, including older people themselves) that would provide for the well-being of the elderly in all walks of life, taking into account that the aged are not a homogeneous group and creating opportunities for individual choices.

20. Expansion of research projects and facilities and provision for the utilization of research findings as soon as possible in planning and development of social-welfare programs and services.

21. Development of new, and improvement of existing, educational and training programs for professionals, paraprofessionals, nonprofessionals, and volunteers working with the elderly, linking the formal with the informal network of services.

22. Development of a system whereby the existence of projects can be readily communicated to the public and where the results of successful demonstration projects can be made part of programs and services as quickly as possible.[5]

Baum and Baum have examined, in their cross-cultural study *Growing Old, a Societal Perspective*, what the modern fate of being old entails, in contrast to previous periods in human history.[6] They conclude that the modern fate of being old is a fourfold experience: (1) a self-perpetuating form of intergenerational solidarity in economic or material care; (2) a self-perpetuating intergenerational solidarity in political bonds of citizenship; (3) abandonment in the areas of spiritual care; and (4) death as a liberation from the uncertainties in the human condition. In other words, growing old evokes solidarity among generations and assures a bond of continuity, linking the past with the present to a future; it also leads to abandonment when people die and leave others behind to come to terms with themselves as autonomous human beings; however, death also liberates and makes the uncertainties of the human condition certain and thereby, predictably, provides a boundary that forces a search for meaning to our journey in this world.

Social policy, then, can also be perceived as a continuous process of searching out guideposts for a meaningful existence that assures people of not merely existential security but also existential fulfillment as human beings in the family of all people all over the world, young and old, black and white, Gentile and Jew, brother and sister. To strive toward such a vision is a continuing task that knows no boundaries, no end, and no beginning: it is an eternal and a timeless struggle for social justice and human caring, a combining of the Judaeic concept of *Tzedokah* and the Christian ideal of *caritas*!

Notes

1. Neil Gilbert and Harry Specht, *Dimensions of Social Welfare Policy* (Englewood, N.J.: Prentice-Hall, 1974).

2. John Rawls, *Social Justice* (Cambridge, Mass.: Harvard University Press, 1974).

3. Howard E. Freeman and Clarence C. Sherwood, *Social Research and Social Policy* (Englewood Cliffs, N.J.: Prentice-Hall, 1970), p. 3.

4. Louis Lowy, *Social Work with the Aging: The Challenge and Promise of the Later Years* (New York: Harper & Row, 1979), chap. 14.

5. Louis Lowy, "Social Welfare and the Aging," in *Understanding Aging* ed. Marian Spencer and Josephine Dorr (New York: Appleton-Century-Crofts, 1975).

6. Martha Baum and Rainer C. Baum, *Growing Old: A Societal Perspective* (Englewood Cliffs, N.J.: Prentice-Hall, 1980), chap. 8.

2 The Graying of America

The Report by the Special Committee on Aging of the United States Senate *Developments in Aging, 1978* begins its chapter "Every Ninth American" with the following statement:

> When we declared our independence, every 50th American was a so-called older person (aged 65-plus). They came to some 50,000 out of an estimated total population of 2.5 million or 2 percent.
>
> By the beginning of this century, the numbers of older persons had increased more rapidly than the young and represented every 25th American.
>
> At the beginning of 1979, the estimated 24.4 million older Americans made up just over 11 percent of the population—"Every Ninth American."
>
> But something quite different with new potentials for study and concern is also becoming evident. In the past, since the proportion of older persons in the population grew somewhat faster than did the other age groups, we had a growing total population, including the aged. The recent trends, however, have been different. The fertility rates since the end of the postwar baby boom have actually been below zero population growth so that continuation and the passage of time will bring us an aging society with an increasing median age.
>
> Even cursory consideration indicates the implications for shifting of product markets, clothing styles, social and recreational facilities, types of housing, health care facilities, entertainment, et cetera.[1]

Demographic Changes

The elderly population has been growing much faster than the nation's population as a whole during the twentieth century and can be expected to continue growing at a rapid rate until the first third of the next century. Associated with this past growth have been changes in the social and economic structure of our society, particularly those aspects that affect the elderly. Massive public programs such as social security and medicare have been launched and now provide benefits to nearly every person 65 and older, as well as many under 65 The average retirement age has been declining, allowing the newly retired to spend additional years in the pursuit of leisure and other noncareer activities. About one million persons 60 years of age and older reside in over twenty-four thousand nursing homes.

The forces that have shaped the demographic structure of our society, particularly the increasing number and proportion of elderly, are well known. Except for the "baby boom" following World War II, fertility rates have been steadily declining. At the same time, medical advances, especially those that have drastically reduced infant and maternal mortality, have added about twenty-six years to the average life span since 1900. Although the average life expectancy for persons at age 60 has not increased as dramatically, many more persons are now surviving to that age. Immigration from abroad brought about 17 million (primarily young) persons to this country in the first quarter of this century but has been at a relatively low level for decades. The survivors of the turn-of-the-century waves of immigration are now elderly, as are many of their children.

The elderly population increased in size from 4.9 million in 1900 to nearly seven times this number in 1977 (32.8 million), (see table 2-1) and the population under 60 years of age increased at only one-fourth this rate. Current Census Bureau projections indicate that the elderly will continue to grow at a faster pace than the rest of the population into the twenty-first century. The growth rate for the elderly population will slow somewhat around the turn of the next century as the relatively smaller cohorts who were born during the Depression of the 1930s reach the age of 60. However, as persons born during the baby-boom years reach the age of 60 early in the next century, most of the growth in the nation's population will occur in the older age brackets. Between 1977 and 2035, the total population is projected to grow by about 40 percent, from 217 million to 304 million persons. The elderly population is projected to more than double in size during this same period, from 33 to 71 million persons.[2]

As a result of these demographic changes, the average age of our population has risen from 23 years to over 29 years since 1900, and it is projected to climb to 38 years by the year 2035. At the beginning of this century, persons 60 years old and over represented one of every sixteen persons. They now represent one of every seven and, by the year 2035, will represent about one-fourth of the total population. Among the population 25 years old and over, the elderly now represent one-fourth of this age group and will represent over one-third by the year 2035.

Beyond the sheer growth in the numbers of elderly, the demographic and socioeconomic characteristics of this population also have undergone considerable change in the past and will continue to change dramatically in the future (see tables 2-2 and 2-3). For example, the elderly population has become increasingly "older." The size of the population 60 and over has increased nearly seven times since 1900, but the population 75 and over has experienced a tenfold increase and the 85-and-over age group has grown by about seventeen times. Currently, about one-fourth of the elderly population is 75 and over, and this proportion is projected to increase to over one-

Table 2-1
Estimated Population 65 and Older, by State (1977)

State	Number (thousands)	Percent of Total Population	Percent Increase 1970-1977	Percent below Poverty Level, 1975[a]
Alabama	398	10.8	22.6	31.6
Alaska	9	2.3	36.9	5.0
Arizona	250	10.9	55.3	12.2
Arkansas	285	13.3	20.3	29.1
California	2,185	10.0	21.9	7.6
Colorado	224	8.6	19.7	14.1
Connecticut	340	10.9	18.2	7.8
Delaware	53	9.2	22.0	12.6
District of Columbia	71	10.3	1.2	13.6
Florida	1,444	17.1	46.5	11.3
Georgia	456	9.0	24.8	31.9
Hawaii	63	7.1	43.5	9.7
Idaho	84	9.7	23.9	15.1
Illinois	1,194	10.6	9.6	10.2
Indiana	554	10.4	12.6	11.0
Iowa	374	13.0	7.0	12.6
Kansas	293	12.6	10.5	12.2
Kentucky	382	11.0	13.6	22.6
Louisiana	363	9.3	19.0	29.3
Maine	130	12.0	13.7	14.7
Maryland	359	8.7	20.5	11.4
Massachusetts	687	11.9	8.4	5.9
Michigan	850	9.3	13.3	9.0
Minnesota	454	11.4	11.4	12.8
Mississippi	266	11.1	20.1	37.0
Missouri	622	12.9	11.3	16.9
Montana	79	10.4	15.3	13.3
Nebraska	199	12.8	9.2	15.4
Nevada	51	8.0	64.4	7.3
New Hampshire	93	11.0	19.6	9.9
New Jersey	808	11.0	16.5	8.2
New Mexico	98	8.2	39.1	19.5
New York	2,082	11.6	6.7	9.1
North Carolina	530	9.6	28.7	24.7
North Dakota	77	11.7	16.0	15.4
Ohio	1,110	10.4	11.7	11.3
Oklahoma	349	12.4	16.8	22.1
Oregon	274	11.5	21.6	11.4
Pennsylvania	1,432	12.1	13.0	11.1
Rhode Island	118	12.6	13.7	13.6
South Carolina	247	8.6	30.3	26.8

Table 2-1 *(cont.)*

State	Number (thousands)	Percent of Total Population	Percent Increase 970-1977	Percent Below Poverty Level, 1975[a]
South Dakota	88	12.7	9.2	17.1
Tennessee	465	10.8	21.6	26.0
Texas	1,228	9.6	24.3	22.5
Utah	98	7.7	27.0	13.3
Vermont	54	11.1	13.5	15.3
Virginia	454	8.8	24.1	18.2
Washington	386	10.6	20.5	9.8
West Virginia	219	11.8	13.0	19.4
Wisconsin	534	11.5	13.4	8.6
Wyoming	35	8.6	15.6	13.2
Total	23,494	10.9	17.6	14.0

Source: U.S. Department of Health, Education and Welfare, Office of Human Development Services, *Facts about Older Americans* (Washington, D.C., 1978), DHEW Publication (OHDS) 79-20006, pp. 2-4.

[a]Data exclude persons in institutions.

third by the year 2035. The 85 + group now constitutes one of every sixteen elderly persons; by 2035, they will represent one of every ten. These increases in the older age groups will add about three years to the median age of the 60 + population, from 69 years in 1977 to 72 years in 2035.[3]

Where Do Older Americans Live?

In 1977, about half (45 percent) of persons 65 + lived in seven states. California and New York had over 2 million, and Florida, Illinois, Ohio, Pennsylvania, and Texas had over 1 million. Since 1970, the 65 + group in seven states has grown by more than 30 percent: Nevada (64 percent), Arizona (55 percent), Florida (47 percent), Hawaii (44 percent), New Mexico (39 percent), Alaska (37 percent), and South Carolina (30 percent), and the 65 + group was 12 percent or more of the total population in eleven states: Florida (17.1 percent), Arkansas (13.3 percent), Iowa (13.0 percent), Missouri (12.9 percent), Nebraska (12.8 percent), South Dakota (12.7 percent), Kansas and Rhode Island (12.6 percent), Oklahoma (12.4 percent), Pennsylvania (12.1 percent), and Maine (12.0 percent). There were eleven states in which over one-fifth of persons 65 + were below the poverty level in 1975: Mississippi (37.0 percent), Georgia (31.9 percent), Alabama (31.6 percent), Louisiana (29.3 percent), Arkansas (29.1 percent), South Carolina (26.8 percent), Tennessee (26.0 percent), North Carolina (24.7 percent),

Table 2-2

Number of Persons of All Ages and 60 Years and Older (1900 and 1977) and Projections for 2000 and 2035

Subject	All Ages	60+ Total	60 to 64	65+ Total	65 to 74	75+	85+
Number (in thousands)							
Total							
1900	76,212	4,879	1,795	3,084	2,189	895	122
1977	216,745	32,793	9,362	23,431	14,577	8,853	2,040
2000	260,378	41,973	10,151	31,822	17,436	14,386	3,756
2035	304,486	70,514	14,709	55,805	29,627	26,178	6,854
Female							
1900	37,243	2,401	875	1,526	1,070	456	68
1977	111,071	18,868	4,983	13,885	8,251	5,634	1,394
2000	133,790	24,451	5,346	19,105	9,762	9,341	2,693
2035	158,184	41,086	7,716	33,370	16,519	16,851	4,913
Nonwhite							
1900	9,344	448	172	276	185	91	na
1977	29,009	3,048	881	2,167	1,420	747	195
2000	41,464	4,991	1,324	3,667	2,216	1,450	392
2035	57,509	12,275	2,888	9,387	5,344	4,043	1,049
Percent Change for Selected Periods							
Total							
1900 to 1977	184.4	572.1	421.6	659.8	565.9	889.2	1,572.1
1977 to 2000	20.1	28.0	8.4	35.8	19.6	62.5	84.1
2000 to 2035	16.9	68.0	44.9	75.4	69.9	82.0	82.5
1977 to 2035	40.5	115.0	57.1	138.2	103.2	195.7	236.0
Female							
1900 to 1977	198.2	685.8	469.5	809.9	671.1	1,135.5	1,950.0
1977 to 2000	20.5	29.6	7.3	37.6	18.3	65.8	93.2
2000 to 2035	18.2	68.0	44.3	74.7	69.2	80.4	82.4
1977 to 2035	42.4	117.8	54.8	140.3	100.2	199.1	252.4
Nonwhite							
1900 to 1977	210.5	580.4	412.2	685.1	667.6	720.9	na
1977 to 2000	42.9	63.7	50.3	69.2	56.1	94.1	101.0
2000 to 2035	38.7	145.9	118.1	156.0	141.2	178.8	167.6
1977 to 2035	98.2	302.7	227.8	333.2	276.3	441.2	437.9

Source: Bureau of the Census, various publications, and unpublished data.
na: not available.

Kentucky (22.6 percent), Texas (22.5 percent), and Oklahoma (22.1 percent). Finally, about 31 percent of the elderly lived outside the nation's metropolitan areas in 1976, compared with 26 percent of all other age groups.[4]

Table 2-3
Percentage Distribution of Persons of All Ages and 60 Years and Older (1900 and 1977) and Projections for 2000 and 2035

Subject	All Ages	60+ Total	60 to 64	65+ Total	65 to 74	75+	85+
All Ages							
Total							
1900	100.0	6.4	2.4	4.0	2.9	1.2	0.2
1977	100.0	15.1	4.3	10.8	6.7	4.1	0.9
2000	100.0	16.1	3.9	12.2	6.7	5.5	1.4
2035	100.0	23.2	4.8	18.3	9.7	8.6	2.3
Female							
1900	100.0	6.4	2.3	4.1	2.9	1.2	0.2
1977	100.0	17.0	4.5	12.5	7.4	5.1	1.3
2000	100.0	18.3	4.0	14.3	7.3	7.0	2.0
2035	100.0	26.0	4.9	21.1	10.4	10.7	3.1
Nonwhite							
1900	100.0	4.8	1.8	3.0	2.0	1.0	na
1977	100.0	10.5	3.0	7.5	4.9	2.6	0.7
2000	100.0	12.0	3.2	8.8	5.3	3.5	0.9
2035	100.0	21.3	5.0	16.3	9.3	7.0	1.8
60 Years and Older							
Total							
1900	x	100.0	36.8	63.2	44.9	18.3	2.5
1977	x	100.0	28.5	71.5	44.5	27.0	6.2
2000	x	100.0	24.2	75.8	41.5	34.3	8.9
2035	x	100.0	20.9	79.1	42.0	37.1	9.7
Female							
1900	x	100.0	36.4	63.6	44.6	19.0	2.8
1977	x	100.0	26.4	73.6	43.7	29.9	7.4
2000	x	100.0	21.9	78.1	39.9	38.2	11.0
2035	x	100.0	18.8	81.2	40.2	41.0	12.0
Nonwhite							
1900	x	100.0	38.4	61.6	41.3	20.3	na
1977	x	100.0	28.9	71.1	46.6	24.5	6.4
2000	x	100.0	26.5	73.5	44.4	29.1	7.9
2035	x	100.0	23.5	76.5	43.5	32.9	8.5

Source: Bureau of the Census, various publications, and unpublished data.
na: not available; x: not applicable.

Women

Women now constitute a much larger proportion of the elderly population than in the past. In 1900, elderly men actually outnumbered women by a slight margin. However, the medical advances in this century have had a greater impact on the health of women, particularly during the child-bearing years. The average life expectancy of white women increased by 26 years between 1900 and 1975; for white men, the increase was only 21 years. Based on 1975 mortality rates, white female children can expect to live 77 years on the average, about 8 years longer than white males. The increase in life expectancy at age 60 since 1900 has been greater for white women than for white men (6.7 versus 2.4 years). White women who were 60 years old in 1975 could expect to live an additional 22 years, about 5 years longer than white males of the same age.

One experience that most elderly women will eventually have in common is the loss of their husband. The vast majority of women in their younger adult years are married, but fewer than half of all women 60 years old and over are currently living with their spouse. Among the noninstitutional population, the number of elderly widows (7.9 million in 1976) slightly exceeds the number of elderly wives (7.8 million), and the rate of widowhood rises from only 23 percent for women 60 to 64 years to 70 percent for those 75 years and older. A report on elderly widows stated that ". . . the conditions of their existence are considerably different from the elderly population in general. Most widows live alone on relatively low incomes. One-fourth rely on cash incomes below the Federal Government's poverty index. Many have given up their homes and moved to smaller apartments, but housing costs consume a large share of their income. Most do not have automobiles and must rely on other sources of transportation."[5] There are an additional half million elderly widows living in nursing homes. These widows constitute over one-half of the nursing-home population and three-fourths of all elderly women in these institutions. Clearly, future growth in the number of elderly women will increase the number of elderly who will require a variety of supportive services to cope with such difficulties as living alone in declining health and with low incomes.

Nonwhites

Just as this century's medical advances have had a larger impact on women than men, these advances have had a greater impact on blacks and persons of other races as compared to white persons. Average life expectancy at birth for white persons increased by nearly one-half between 1900 and 1975, but it doubled for persons of races other than white. The increase in life expectancy at age 60 was also greater for nonwhites than for whites. As a result of this and other demographic factors, persons or races other than white are projected to grow in number about 300 percent by 2035 (compared to 115 percent for all races), increasing their proportion of the elderly population from about one-tenth today to one-sixth in the year 2035.

In the near future, then, the elderly in general and the older elderly in particular will continue to grow in numbers at a more rapid rate than the population as a whole. Associated with this numerical change will be changes in the socioeconomic characteristics of the elderly. However, the segments of the elderly population that will be growing most rapidly (the oldest of the old, women, and persons of races other than white) will be the same groups that have suffered more from such common problems of the elderly as poor health, social isolation, and poverty.[6]

Elderly Living Alone

One of the most striking phenomena that have occurred in recent decades has been the rapid growth in the number of elderly who live alone. Since 1960, the number living alone has increased three times as fast as one would have predicted from the simple growth in the size of the elderly population. The proportion living alone has increased from one-sixth of all noninstitutionalized elderly in 1960 to one-fourth in 1976, and the number has risen from 3.8 million in the earlier year to 7.9 million in the latter year. The trend toward living alone has been particularly noticeable among elderly women and the oldest subgroups of the elderly population. Although the number of elderly men living alone grew by 600,000, or 56 percent, between 1960 and 1976, the proportion living alone in 1976 was not much higher than in 1960 (13 percent versus 11 percent). However, the number of elderly women maintaining households by themselves grew by 3.5 million or 132 percent during this sixteen-year period, and the proportion living alone rose from 22 percent to 35 percent. Likewise, the increase in single-person households among persons 75 years old and over far outstripped the rates for the younger elderly, being twice as high as the rate for the 65-to-74 age group and three times that of the 60-to-64 age group. In 1976, over one-third (37 percent) of all persons 75 and older lived alone, and nearly one-half (48 percent) of all women in this age group resided alone.

There are many contributing factors to this trend toward living alone among the elderly. One of the principal factors, of course, is the increasingly longer life span of women compared to men, coupled with the fact that most women are generally younger than their husbands. Most wives outlive their husbands by several years. Few elderly widows remarry, and most of them (about two-thirds) live alone. The disparity between the number of elderly widows and the number of elderly widowers has grown since 1930 from a ratio of about 2 to 1 to over 5 to 1. Other factors contributing to the increase in living alone include: (1) greater financial security because of new income and health-care-support programs (for example, supplemental security income, medicare), as well as automatic cost-of-living increases in social security benefits and wider coverage under private pension plans; (2) the increasing geographic dispersal of families due to rising levels of education, occupational mobility, and improvemen. in communication and transportation; and (3) smaller family size; most of today's elderly were in their child-bearing years before World War II, when birth rates were relatively low, and therefore they have fewer children than earlier generations.

Future changes in these other factors could cause a slowing or reversal of the trend toward living alone among the elderly in the next few decades. For example, the parents of the baby-boom generation, who are currently beginning to join the ranks of the 60-and-older population, will have larger families to rely on when residential-relocation decisions must be made. Future periods of high inflation or a continuation of the current energy and housing shortages could undermine the desirability or economic feasibility of living alone. Nevertheless, elderly persons with the highest rates of living alone (women and the oldest of the elderly) are the same groups that will be growing at the most rapid rates in the future. Even if the rate of increase in living alone slows somewhat, it appears that the number of elderly living alone will continue to climb.[7]

Changes in Characteristics of the Elderly

Many of the changes that have occurred in the social and economic structure of the United States are reflected in the characteristics of the elderly population only after a delay of years or even decades. For example, the advent of universal education and the changing values of our society regarding the benefits of higher education have been reflected in the constant rise in the median number of years of school completed. Between 1940 (the first year for which such data are available) and 1976, the median for persons 25 years old and over rose steadily from 8.6 to 12.4 years. For elderly persons, who received most of their education during or before the Depression of the 1930s, the median number of school years remained at slightly over 8 years for the decades between 1940 and 1960. Since 1960, the median for the elderly has risen from 8.3 to 10.3 years, and this figure can be expected to rise to 12 years around the year 1990. Although the overall median for the elderly population was 10.3 in 1976, this figure ranged from 12 years for the 60-to-64 age group to about 9 years for persons 75 and over.

Related to the increase in educational attainment is the decrease in the number of elderly persons with language difficulties. Although consistent data on languages spoken by the population are not available, data on the number of elderly persons who were born in foreign countries can at least indicate the likely direction of the trend. According to the decennial censuses conducted since 1900, the number of persons 60 years old and older who were born abroad increased steadily from about 1.5 million at the turn of the century to 4.2 million in 1960, a result of the aging of the large number of pre-World War I immigrants. Between 1960 and 1970 this number declined from 4.2 million to 3.7 million, and it will continue to decline in the future. Although the number of foreign-born elderly rose between 1900 and 1960, their proportion of the entire elderly population declined steadily from one-third in 1900 to one-seventh in 1970. This proportion will decline at an accelerating rate in the coming years, reaching one of every twenty during the 1980s. As noted, not all the foreign-born elderly have difficulty with the English language. However, a survey conducted in 1975 by the Bureau of the Census indicated that 5 percent or 1 million persons 65 years old and older usually spoke a language other than English The usual speaking language for half of these persons was either Spanish (30 percent) or Italian (20 percent).

In addition to educational attainment, the occupational history of the elderly population is also changing. In the last several decades, the occupational structure of the nation's labor force has undergone a considerable transformation. Many occupations have flourished, particularly those in the professions, sciences, public services, and others that generally require higher levels of education and that return a high level of earnings. Entire industries have been created or have experienced phenomenal growth rates, for example, aerospace and computer technology, electronics, and telecommunications. On the other hand, many occupations, particularly farming and unskilled labor, have lost much of their former share of the labor force.

As with education, the full extent of these changes in the nation's occupational structure are not yet reflected in the occupational histories of today's elderly. To illustrate, let us compare the occupational distributions of employed males who were 35 to 44 years old in 1970 (all of whom will be over 60 by the year 1990) with a similar group as of 1950 (the survivors of whom were 62 to 71 years old in 1977). During this twenty-year period, the proportion of these workers who were employed in white-collar jobs rose from 33 percent to 44 percent, most of the increase occurring in the highly paid professional and technical occupations (8 percent in 1950 to 17 percent in 1970). The proportion of workers in blue-collar jobs remained about the same (49 percent and 47 percent, respectively). However, the proportion engaged in unskilled labor or farm work declined from 20 percent in 1950 to only 8 percent in 1970. Thus, the occupational history of tomorrow's elderly retired population will be considerably different from today's elderly. In fact, some of America's first astronauts will reach their sixty-first birthday in the next five years.

One of the effects of these changes in the characteristics of the elderly has been to increase the average income of older persons and decrease the number whose incomes fell below the poverty level. Other factors that have contributed to the relative as well as absolute improvement in the

economic situation of the elderly population have been the general movement of the economy in recent years, the increasing coverage of the elderly
under a variety of public and private pension plans, and the implementation of new income-support programs for the elderly. Some of the income-
support programs include supplemental security income, medicare, food
stamps, and housing subsidies. In addition, large increases in benefit levels
and a cost-of-living escalator clause have been enacted for the social
security program.

During the 1960s, a period of economic progress for the population as a
whole, the income of both younger and older families and individuals rose
at similar rates. After adjustment for inflation between 1960 and 1970, the
median income of families headed by persons 65 years and older rose by 33
percent and the median income for persons 65 years and older who lived
alone rose by 41 percent. The 1970s have been much more difficult years for
the economy. The unemployment rate more than doubled between 1969 and
1976 (3.5 percent versus 7.7 percent). At the same time, the cost of living (as
measured by the consumer price index) rose by 55 percent, as compared to
only 24 percent between 1960 and 1969. The effects of this downturn in the
economy were felt more strongly by younger families and individuals than
by the elderly. The median income of younger families and individuals (25
to 64 years of age) grew by only 4 percent each between 1970 and 1976,
whereas the income of families and individuals 65 years and older grew by
18 percent and 22 percent, respectively.

The trend in the number of persons with incomes below the federal
government's poverty index was similar to the trend in median income.
During the 1960s, large decreases in the number of poor were experienced
by all age groups. Between 1969 and 1976, the number of persons under 60
who were below the poverty level increased from 18.3 to 20.7 million. For
persons 60 and older, however, the number of poor continued to decline,
from 5.9 million in 1969 to 4.3 million in 1976. These 4.3 million elderly
poor represented one-seventh of all noninstitutionalized persons 60 years
and older.

Although the number of elderly poor declined by 1.6 million in recent
years, this decline was partially offset by an increase of 400 thousand in the
number of elderly persons with incomes above the poverty level but below
the "near-poor" level. In addition, the subgroup of the elderly population
that exhibited the greatest decline in poverty during the 1970s consisted of
elderly males living with their wives or other family members. The
subgroups that experienced slower rates of decline in poverty or no decline
at all were the same subgroups that were growing in size most rapidly and
are projected to continue growing at rapid rates: females, minorities, and
those who live alone. These subgroups, women and minorities in particular,
tend to have worked less in the past and to have worked in lower-paying oc-

cupations than white males, and therefore they tend to have fewer financial assets to rely on after retirement.

It is quite difficult to predict future economic trends because of the large number of variables involved. It may well be, however, that the continued rapid rate of growth of these subgroups will insure the continued existence of a substantial number of elderly persons with incomes near or below the poverty level. To illustrate this point, if the age, sex, and race distribution of the elderly population in 1975 had been the same as that projected for the year 2035, the mean income of elderly persons in 1975 would have been about one-tenth lower than was actually reported.

Nevertheless, it is likely that the income and other financial resources of most of the future elderly will be greater than for today's elderly. Tomorrow's elderly will be more highly educated and will have worked in higher-paying occupations. In addition to social security benefits, many will receive pension benefits. A higher proportion of elderly women in the future will have participated in the labor force for a significant number of their preretirement years and will therefore be receiving retirement benefits of their own. Hopefully, the elimination of inequities between the economic situation of whites on the one hand and minority racial and ethnic groups on the other will occur and will be translated into economic security for the future minority elderly.

Regardless of their economic situation, all these data indicate that the elderly population will be both growing rapidly and changing rapidly. If the present trend toward early retirement coupled with longer life expectancy continues, this would mean many more years of retirement. The increasing proportion of elderly who will fall in the 75 + and 85 + age groups will require additional resources to handle the physical and emotional problems that occur more frequently in these age groups. The growing proportion of women, many of whom will be widowed and living alone, will require additional resources to meet the social needs of this subgroup. The rising numbers of elderly who live alone will require housing alternatives to institutionalization so that they may continue to live independent lives while learning to cope with the physical infirmities of their age. The nation's population as a whole, as it becomes progressively older in composition, must learn to deal with the changing needs of its members.[8]

It seems safe to assume that a country with a larger proportion of older people will need less baby food, toys, teachers, and maternity wards. Conversely, demands should rise for retirement homes, medical care, recreational facilities, and entertainment suiting the tastes of the elderly. Political styles too may be altered, since the elderly will have close to one-third of the vote.

Such concerns have spawned much talk of altering the "entry" and "exit" ages for workers. Some have suggested earlier retirement to make way for the young, but others talk about postponing it because men and women will live longer with health intact. In April 1978 mandatory retirement for employment in the private and public sector was advanced from age 65 to 70 by law.

A less tangible concern is that an older society might be less creative, less innovative, more conservative. Without the pressure of large waves of young people, it is argued, a society would become gray and dreary. Critics of this theory say that countries with older populations, like Sweden, Norway, and West Germany are not particularly conservative.

Of greater immediate concern is the matter of dependency. A stable population would have the same proportion of people in the working ages (18 to 65), compared to the dependent young and old, as it does today—about three workers to every two dependents. However, the preponderance of dependents would shift to the elderly group, who are far more costly to care for than the young.

Today, the United States provides relatively poorly for retired people. What will happen when their number doubles? In 1972 a report to the Commission of Population Growth and the American Future of the UN Statistical Office put it this way: "To worry about the supposed behavioral consequence of an aging, or more aged population, is to divert attention from the real issue: how to incorporate a higher proportion of old people into society in a socially and emotionally meaningful way." The graying of America has given Robert N. Butler, director of the National Institute on Aging, reason to hope that "this may be the time when humankind uses a little forethought."

Notes

1. Herman B. Brotman, "The Graying of Every Tenth American or Every Ninth American," in U.S., 95th Congress, 2nd session, Senate, *Developments in Aging, 1978 Report to the Special Committee on Aging, 1978*, pp. xv-xxvi.

2. Ibid., p. xxxiii.

3. U.S. Bureau of Census, *Current Population Reports*, ser. P-20, no. 338 and earlier reports, ser. P-23, nos. 57 and 59; ser. P-23, no. 800; and ser. P-80, nos. 118, 119.

4. U.S. Department of Health, Education and Welfare Office of Human Development Services, *Facts about Older Americans 1978*, DHEW Publication (OHDS) 79-20006 (Washington, D.C., 1978).

5. U.S. Department of Health, Education and Welfare, Administration on Aging, "Elderly Widows," *Statistical Memo*, no. 33 (July 1976):5.

6. U.S. Bureau of the Census, *Current Population Reports*, ser. P-25, nos. 519, 724, and 800.

7. U.S. Department of Health, Education and Welfare, *Facts about Older Americans*.

8. U.S. Bureau of the Census, *Current Population Reports*, ser. P-25, nos. 519, 724, and 800. See also Louis Lowy, *Social Work with the Aging, the Challenge and Promise of the Later Years* (New York: Harper & Row, 1979), pp. 21-40.

3 Toward a National Policy on Aging: The Foundations of Public Social Policy

The phenomenon of aging, with its ensuing personal, social, and political consequences, has received more formal attention by public policy makers in the last decade than at any previous period. One way of achieving a more realistic understanding of age-related issues is through the explicit statement of values and the provision of empirical data in a format useful for the formulation of human-services policy. This will allow policy shaping and policy making to be based on an understanding of values as well as factual understanding about the problems and needs of the elderly population.

Federal and state policy makers across the country point to the inadequacy of their current information base for policy-making needs.[1] In addition, the use of different information sources by various decision makers involved in the social-policy process precludes a systematic understanding of the problems of the elderly population. Service-delivery personnel rely more heavily on information generated from direct contact with older people than do legislators and administrative agency heads, and administrative heads place more emphasis on information from government reports than do service-delivery personnel and legislators.

Some Basic Assumptions

The needs of future older people will differ from the needs of today's elders. As stated in chapter 2 the present generation of elders, particularly the older ones, tends to have low income, low educational achievement, low expectations for services, and relatively low political sophistication. Future generations of elders will have higher incomes, higher educational achievement, higher expectation for services, and greater political sophistication. Everyone who will become 65 between now and 2040 is alive today and is being influenced by current events.

Just as growing old is a continuous process beginning at birth and concluding at death, becoming an older person does not represent a sudden break from one's earlier self. A person's distinctive characteristics, abilities, and desires persist in a context of changing needs and times. Therefore the elderly population should be an integral part of society, not a distinct subgroup differing from all others. Elders share needs with other groups in society and should be fully integrated into community life.

The elderly population is heterogeneous. There are younger and older, rich and poor elders, there are activists and nonactivists, healthy and ill, satisfied and dissatisfied. Policy making for the elderly must recognize this heterogeneity.

Elements related to satisfaction among elders are, in order of importance: income, living with a spouse, health status, and education. These elements, obviously, must be a focus of attention for policy makers.

Societal attitudes and stereotypes affect society's policies toward the elderly. The need to eliminate and change negative attitudes and stereotypes is obvious.

There are at least four important characteristics of the elderly population that pose a special challenge:

1. There are the young-old (60 to 75) and the old-old (75 and older). The old-old are the fastest growing segment of the elderly population and will continue to be so. Large numbers of old-older people pose new sets of problems for social policy.

2. The male-female ratio is changing. Presently there are 144 women over 65 to every 100 men. Of the old-old, the ratio is even more dramatic. Planning for the old-old is primarily planning for the needs of older women.

3. There are the poor who become old and the old who become poor. The latter must cope with a vastly altered life-style, which may have negative social, psychological, and personal consequences. For the former, old age is the final insult and hardship added to what may have been a lifetime of inadequate income, inadequate health care, and demoralization.

4. The proportion of minority elderly is increasing. Between 1960 and 1970, the number of all elderly persons over 75 grew by 28.6 percent; at the same time the nonwhite elderly in this group grew 76.1 percent.

Federal, state, and local responsibilities for the elderly will continue to evolve. It is increasingly expected that income maintenance and the payment for health care will become federal responsibilities and states will be the primary social- and health-service providers, with actual service delivery occurring on the local level.

What are public policies? Morris defines public policies as:

> guides as to the aims of governing to which priorities are assigned and to the means which are acceptable to, or preferred by, a particular government. These guides are general, in that they indicate which problems a government will choose to deal with and which way a government will choose to move when it is confronted with the necessity to take action. In this sense, then, policies are guiding principles for a government. A government may choose a general policy of stressing its citizens' domestic well-being over acquisition of power in foreign affairs. When the well-being depends upon control over external sources, the policy choice is whether

to concentrate on domestic resources alone or not. Within such a general policy, a government must decide to what extent it will regulate the acts of its citizens in order to pursue the goal of general well-being, to what extent it will direct its citizens to act in their private capacities to satisfy their own needs; or to what extent it will provide for its citizens' needs directly through government agencies.[2]

But policy is not only general, applying to all of government and all of society; it is also specific and sectorial, as some policy may only affect a segment of that society, as, in this discussion, the aging population.

Social policies are affected by the demographic composition, by the level of productivity of a society (be it an industrialized, a preindustrial, or a developing country), by the way the social structure operates, by assumptions made about human nature, by the historical legacy of that society, and, last but not least, by ideologies and value assumptions extant in a society. Policies that social institutions produce reflect the dominance of some values over others, and social problems are defined according to normative conceptions and the degree of tenacity in which they are held. These value choices and definitions of problems are not necessarily derived from agreements by members of that society, nor are they the result of compromises or statements among those persons most affected by them. As we know, societies are unequal in terms of resources to which members have access and the powers that can be brought to bear by various groups and classes. And some classes and social groupings are in a better position than others to influence a definition of social problems or a determination of social priorities. The aged, for example, may attempt to influence social priorities and resultant public policies, but they are only one of a number of other groups competing for determination of the various priorities and policy choices open to them.

Values, Knowledge, and Power

Values and ideologies prevailing in a society, the knowledge and data base about a particular population and its needs or problems, and the power relationships influence, if not shape, social policies. Let us briefly examine these factors with respect to the aging.

Values

American society is characterized by a dominant value orientation that emphasizes doing rather than being, the present and future rather than the past, independence rather than dependence or interdependence.[3] An attitude can be defined as an individual's characteristic way of regarding an object, person, or process. Attitudes are developed in individuals as part of the socialization process, and they significantly influence not only an individual's perception of the external world but also an individual's perception of self. Attitudes held about old age and older people are no exception and dominate the experience of growing old in our society.

Attitudes can be conceptualized as having three components: cognition, affect, and action. For example, in the attitude "the elderly cohort is a surplus population," the cognitive component is the perception of elderly individuals as unneeded and, consequently, having little value to society. One of the major problems of the elderly is that they have been an invisible minority. Not being perceived by society has resulted in a lack of attention to the needs, problems, and strengths of the elderly.

The affectual, that is, emotional, component will vary for each individual. In the instance of an elderly person perceiving the elderly as having little value, the affectual response would be a significant lowering of self-worth. On the other hand, the affectual component would be quite different if a public policy maker had this attitude.

The action component will likewise vary among the different individuals sharing this attitude. The possible action component of an elderly person having this attitude might range from withdrawal from family and friends to, in its most extreme form, suicide. The public policy maker, however, might decide to curtail the number of food stamps provided to the elderly poor or the availability of dental care through medicaid. Action or behavior is undoubtedly influenced by attitudes, but behavior becomes a part of an individual's environment. Behavior as part of the environment is influenced and modified by factors in the environment. Thus the influence on individual attitudes will be modified by a particular setting or milieu.

Existing attitudes always have a profound effect on individuals and society and should be considered an important element of any attempt to modify the situation of the elderly population. Since attitudes are learned responses, they can also be unlearned. For example, the elderly themselves, after experiencing old age, tend to have more positive attitudes about old age than young people[4]; and researchers found that young people who had direct experience with old people saw them more positively than did young people who had little or no direct exposure to old people.[5] Increased participation in society of elderly persons can do much to develop more positive attitudes about aging.

Stereotypes are oversimplified and often inaccurate generalizations that dominate an individual's perception of a specific group. The commonly held stereotypic version of the older population is characteristically unfavorable, including visions of increasing inactivity and disability and decreasing intelligence and sexuality. Such a negative picture is frequently manifested in the interaction between young and old, resulting in rejection and emotional pain.[6]

Ageism, Disengagement, and Its Consequences

Ageism, a term coined by Butler, is defined as "a process of systematic stereotyping of and discrimination against people, because they are old, just as racism and sexism accomplish this with skin color and gender."[7] Ageism complements displays of negative expressions with expressions of the positive values of being young while implying the negative values of being old. Ageism can be seen in statements such as: "she acts so young," or "that picture is beautiful, you paint just like a young person," or "isn't she cute, she thinks so young." According to these statements, certain behavior is appropriate only to the young, including ability such as painting and types of thinking. An implicit element of ageism is the view that the elderly are somehow different from the rest of society and therefore not subject to the same desires, aspirations, concerns, fears, or problems.

A macrocosmic view of the aging experience reveals a pattern of social and psychological disengagement between the aged and many earlier role-related activities.[8] The disengagement theory posits that mutual withdrawal between society and the individual older person is a natural process.[9] Critiques of this theory have refuted many of its aspects and have pointed out that withdrawal is sometimes self-initiated, at other times externally imposed, and does not include all of life's activities.[10] Binstock and Hudson, for example, show that there is, for many elderly, an increase in political activity after retirement and that there is a positive linear relationship between age and political interest.[11] Forced disengagement, which is frequently precipitated by mandatory-retirement policy, spawns a self-fulfilling prophecy.

Most older Americans are not able to enjoy the benefits accompanying a position of solid economic status, since many elderly have only minimal financial resources at their disposal; indeed, many older persons live in poverty. About 15.0 percent or 3.3 million persons 65+ were below the poverty level in 1976. Among elderly whites, one of every eight (13 percent) was poor, but about one-third (35 percent) of elderly blacks and one-fourth (28 percent) of elderly Spanish persons were poor. The proportion below the poverty level was much higher for elderly persons living alone or with nonrelatives (30 percent) than for those living in families (8 percent). Persons 65+ who resided outside the nation's metropolitan areas were more likely to be poor (20 percent) than were elderly metropolitan residents (12 percent). Of the 8.1 million families with a 65+ head, 726,000 or 9 percent were below the poverty level. Most (82 percent) of the income received by families was derived from public sources such as social security, supplemental security, and public assistance. For nonpoor families with a head 65 +, only one-third (34 percent) of the income was from such sources. About 37 percent was received in the form of wages, salaries, and self-employment income.

About two-thirds or 2.1 million of the elderly poor were persons living alone or with nonrelatives. As with elderly families, nearly all (93 percent) the income received by 65 + poor individuals was from public sources. Among nonpoor individuals, only 46 percent of their income was received from such sources. One-seventh (15 percent) was from earnings and about two-fifths (39 percent) was from all other sources. Of the 4.2 million elderly families who received more than half of their income from public sources, only 15 percent were poor. However, about 39 percent of the 5.0 million elderly individuals who received over half of their income from these sources were below the poverty level.[12] (See chapter 4.)

Although the causes of poverty among the elderly are complex, two categories are highly relevant to policy makers—the "old poor," and the "new poor." The former category, the old poor, consists of individuals who have been poor for much of their lives and their old-age poverty is merely an extension of their earlier situation. The cause of poverty for these individuals is not directly related to their age, and future attempts to eliminate this category of poor must incorporate more effective intervention strategies when the individual is younger and more capable of achieving and maintaining an improved economic status. The latter category, the "new poor," consists of eldelry forced, by one reason or another (for example, retirement), to live on a fixed income; the cause of the second category of poor is therefore significantly different than the first. Are these the modern "worthy poor," as the Elizabethan Poor Laws of 1601 would have defined them?

The group that most dramatically experiences age-related poverty is elderly women according to the 1978 U.S. Bureau of the Census Report on "Characteristics of the Low-Income Population"; specifically, these are the elderly women who are either separated (54.5 percent of this group are below the national poverty income level), divorced (31.4 percent of this group are below the national poverty income level), or widowed (24.9 percent of this group are below the national poverty income level). The reason why many of these women find themselves in poverty is that they cannot meet the criteria for receiving standard postretirement benefits, which emphasizes the need for policy makers to examine this critical situation despite some increased welfare benefits through the supplemental security income program. Directly related to income is employment. Public policy facilitates forced withdrawal from employment, often resulting in psychological trauma and other negative consequences to the individuals.

A second consequence of coerced disengagement is residential relocation. Financial realities sometimes cause an elderly person to move unwillingly from his home. Such forced relocation has resulted in a wide variety of negative consequences, ranging from decreased life satisfaction[13] to premature death.[14]

A third, and more subtle, by-product of imposed disengagement is the formation of inappropriate "assigned" roles for the elderly. For example, a common outcome of an elderly person's frequent exposure to an assigned characteristic (dependency, for example) is the acquisition of that characteristic by the elderly individual. This self-fulfilling prophecy also occurs as a result of the interaction to the elderly with public programs: for instance, a program intended to encourage self-sufficiency in fact fosters dependency because of the patronizing treatment given to older people by the providers of services. This is why providers at all levels of the public-policy-service-delivery system must examine the ramifications of their policy decisions and direct interactions with the elderly. By creating an atmosphere of advocacy, support, and education, service organizations such as councils on aging, area agencies, and multiservice centers can more effectively help aging individuals realize their potentials.

The fourth consequence of the social attitudes and policies forcing disengagement is the definition of the elderly as surplus population. This definition is based on the attitudes that the elderly have less potential than the young and are more dependent because they suffer from illness and degeneration—thereby the elderly are defined as being out of the mainstream of society.

Knowledge and Data Base

Increasing accumulation of data, information, and knowledge derived from the biological, behavioral, and social sciences as well as systematized practice experiences from applied fields such as medicine, psychiatry, nursing, social work, and so forth have created and shaped the "new" disciplines of gerontology and geriatrics. These knowledge areas have provided a data base for forging social policies on aging, notably since the 1971 White House Conference.

Social policy toward the aged in our society is of recent origin. After the period of neglect and indifference prior to the 1950s, the first White House conference on aging in 1961 set the stage for consideration of moving toward a national social policy on aging at the second White House conference in 1971. Policy at that time was defined as "a set of focussed, strategically feasible principles and plans for action to provide direction for programs supportive of long-range goals."[15]

In addition to defining the various types of recommendations as guides to policy formulation, the following set of criteria was established for judging the feasibility of a policy proposal: Is it (1) based on known needs of older peoples? (2) consistent with national goals and social values? (3) possible to implement with present knowledge and manpower? (4) realistic in terms of cost? (5) likely to be supported by the general public? Would it (6) benefit the whole community or society as well as just older people? (7) preserve the dignity, freedom, and right of choice of older people? Does it (8) fix responsibility for action on a specific public or private agency or organization?[16] It was expected that rigorous application of these criteria would facilitate the selection of those policies most likely to elicit immedite action, to gain public acceptance, and to find a readiness on the part of society to see them implemented.

Working from this basis, a careful study and evaluation of the circumstances of today's older people and the problems that plague them, even after 20 or more years of effort to improve their conditions, resulted in the selection of fourteen needs areas requiring a more effective set of national policies.

Of the fourteen, nine represent needs areas within which policy and action are required if American society is to be satisfied that its older citizens are to enjoy healthy, active, and meaningful lives. The other five areas, designated as needs-meeting areas, identify the principal means through which action can be brought about—the five needs-meeting areas are the avenues to action for each of the needs.

Schematic Representation of the Relationship
of Needs Areas to Needs-Meeting Areas

Needs-Areas	*Needs-Meeting Areas*
income	planning
health and mental health	training
housing and environment	research and demonstration
nutrition	services, programs, and facilities
education	government and nongovernment
employment and retirement	facilities
retirement roles and activities	
transportation	
spiritual well-being	

In addition to these fourteen needs and needs-meeting areas, a series of eighteen special concerns, such as long-term care of older people, mental-health-care strategies, homemaker-home-health aide services, aging and blindness, Spanish-speaking elderly, the elderly Indian, the aging and aged blacks, the older family, the religious community and the aged, physical and vocational rehabilitation, rural older people, and so forth constituted the substantive part of the conference and formed the basis for recommendations for action by over 3,500 delegates. In the final report, these recommendations were spelled out to lay the groundwork for an American social policy toward the aged.[17]

Social theories are an aid in understanding the needs of individuals and indicate priorities that are necessitated by limited resources. Policies, however, are also influenced by the intentions of legislation, the result of interaction between various pieces of legislation and the way they are enacted, and, finally, by the nature of existing programs.

The history of social programs that benefit the elderly could undoubtedly be traced as far back as the founding of this country, includng such institutions as county homes for the poor and elderly and church food-relief programs. Increasingly, social services have become the responsibility of government, and recently two significant orientations can be detected. On the one hand, social-insurance programs such as social security have been developed for income maintenance, and on the other hand welfare programs have been developed to deal with poverty. The latter are generally service or in-kind programs (medicaid, food stamps, home care, and so on) rather than cash-payment programs. At the same time, there is a growing realization of the importance of keeping individuals out of institutions and in their own communities, which can only be accomplished by comprehensive human services. Such a comprehensive system has not been achieved, and one major obstacle that appears is the result of the conflicting philosophies of income-maintenance and service programs. It is doubtful whether the 1981 White House Conference will come closer to overcoming this obstacle than its predecessor conclave.

Power

Values and knowledge are significant aspects in shaping and directing social policies; however, it is the leverage of power that ultimately forges the decisions that affect the lives of people; it is in the political arena that the multifaceted claims of groups and constituencies are brokered and negotiated. The extent of power held by such groups and their allies determines frequently the direction and content of our social policies.

The emergence of "aging politics" since the early involvements in Milwaukee,[18] the "Ham and Eggs" populist movement, spearheaded by Townsend, to the social security enactment in 1935, has contributed to shaping the "aging agenda" of today.[19] But changes are already in the wings. As Hudson observes:

The aging, long a favored social-welfare constituency in the United States, are in the early stages of being confronted with a series of obstacles which may put their favored status—and its concomitant material and symbolic benefits—in jeopardy. Rapidly rising public policy costs for meeting the needs of an aging population, a nascent but growing reassessment of policy benefits directed toward the elderly, and competitive pressures from other social-welfare constituencies are now threatening two of the aging's longstanding political resources—their singular legitimacy as a policy constituency and their political utility to other actors in the policy process.

These developments hold the clear potential for fundamentally altering old-age politics and policy. The widespread public sympathy and narrower political calculations which have been featured in the passage of many old-age policy enactments will increasingly give way to competitive and cost-based pressures, the effect being to produce a more inclusive and zero-sum politics of aging.[20]

And Robert Binstock poses two questions: (1) Does the aging vote determine the outcome of elections? (2) Do organizations based on aging members and consumers have significant power in conflicts and accommodations taking place in American politics? He answers as follows: "There is no aging vote—no evidence that aging-based appeals can swing a block of older persons' votes. Aging is only one identity among many. Studies show 40-65 percent of the old do not perceive of themselves as old. Most of these are well off, economically and health-wise. Others do not see income, health and housing problems as aging problems."[21]

More recently political scientists speak of the emergence of a younger age group (50 to 65) that could engender greater electoral cohesion based on aging interests. If retirement status becomes a common experience, this group may create a more unified political force that their elders have not formed. Interest groups (involving more than 20 million elderly) have three forms of power: Ready access to public officials—lobbying, and so forth; legitimacy—which gets them public platforms in the national media, at hearings, at the White House conferences, and so on—where they can initiate issues for debate; and electoral bluff, whereby officials who do not want to offend the aged are disposed to favor proposals providing some benefits.

Efforts of these groups are not radical or militant in their attempt to bring about basic changes. They address themselves to two types of policies and programs: direct income-transfer policies and programs (for example, social security and supplemental-security benefits) geared toward obtaining incremental adjustments—a redistribution of wealth rather than major changes; and middleman programs that seek to create new programs—they try to get funds and authority for aging organizations to set up services and facilities for the aged. Summarizing his studies, Binstock writes: "The aging organizations have sufficient power to maintain themselves and their interests, but the goals articulated and sought by these organizations are not suitable to redress fundamentally the economic, biomedical, and social problems of the severely disadvantaged aged—let alone change the general societal status of the aged."[22]

Finally, Hudson, on the subject of future prospects, wrote that:

The political power of the aging, its extent long the subject of debate, will be put to a sterner test than it has faced to this point. The political legitimacy and utility of older persons have always lent a spurious quality to claims which equate the aging's political power with the policy benefits which they have gained. In the coming period, where scrutiny will supplant sympathy, that question should at least be resolved. Success in securing new benefits and maintaining existing ones will depend as never before on the ability of the aging and their organizations to demonstrate that they have the capability of imposing negative sanctions on those who choose not to support them. Costs and competitive pressures combined with the thought that the aging are not to be slighted will put decision-makers in a new and uncomfortable position when it comes to aging issues. Should they choose to continue supporting aging intitiatives, it will be valid testimony to the aging and their organizations having transformed their numbers into an effective political resource.[23]

Foundations of Public Social Policies

As we prepare for the 1981 White House Conference on Aging we are faced with major economic changes in this country, particularly with regard to an increasing scarcity of natural resources, notably energy, and a greater demand on the part of many segments of the population for their share of the natural-resource pie. Therefore we can anticipate that the elderly, who, indeed, have benefitted more than any other age group in the last fifteen years from federal public policies, are likely to be in for a squeeze. Already we notice a backlash by the general population about the claims by the elderly for their share of the public dollar. The prevalence of "ageism" in our society, based on myths, stereotypes, and unfounded assumptions about the aging population, is likely to be increasingly fuelled by this backlash.

The foundations of public policies regarding the aged were laid in 1935 with the passage of the Social Security Act, and its subsequent amendments, that was designed to provide a minimum economic base for a population that was getting older (see chapter 4). The Social Security Act, however, has to be understood within the context of a mandatory-retirement policy from the world of work. Not until 1978 was the arbitrarily fixed age of 65 extended to the likewise arbitrary age of 70. Representative Claude Pepper's efforts to push outward the mandatory-retirement age can be seen as a step in the direction of the full elimination of all mandatory policies.

The most significant legislation for the elderly since the passage of the Social Security Act is the Older Americans Act of 1965 and its subsequent amendments. The act essentially represents an approach to providing social services to the elderly.

Summary of the Older Americans Act

The Older Americans Act was initially passed in 1965 and thereafter amended in 1967, 1969, 1972, 1973, 1975, and again in 1978. The act establishes program objectives and funding to plan, administer, and provide services to meet the special needs of citizens 60 years of age and older (except where the age limit is 55 for community service employment).[24]

The 1978 amendments realign the act into six titles, in contrast to the previous nine. Titles I and II remain substantially unchanged under these amendments, with some new provisions that strengthen the role of the Administration on Aging. Title III consolidates and extends the provisions for social services, senior centers, and nutrition services, previously contained under the old Titles III, V, and VII, which have been repealed. Title IV now contains all provisions for evaluation, research and demonstration, and training project grants. Title V (senior employment) replaces the old Title IX (senior employment). A new Title VI provides for services to Indian tribes.

Title I includes a "Declaration of Objectives," calling for the availability of coordinated, comprehensive programs that include a full range of health, education, and social services for all older citizens who need them. Special priority is given to "the elderly with the greatest economic and social need." Under this title, federal assistance is provided for the planning and operation of such programs developed through a partnership of older citizens, community agencies, and state and local governments.

Title II outlines the structure and role of the federal Administration on Aging (AOA) in the Department of Health, Education and Welfare (DHEW)—now the Department of Health and Human Services (DHHS)—which has overall responsibility for administering programs established under this act and for overseeing and participating in the development of all federal policies and programs affecting the elderly. It provides for a clearinghouse as a central source for all "information related to the needs and interests of older persons," and a Federal Council on Aging to advise the president and the AOA on all federal policies and programs for older Americans.

Title III is the principal source of funding for state and county governments planning for and providing services under this act. As stated, the 1978 amendments expand Title III to include provisions contained in the previous titles III, V, and VII of the Older Americans Act. This new Title III provides for the planning and development of "comprehensive and coordinated service systems," authorizing funding and providing for one administrative structure of three key service areas: social services, (formerly addressed by the old Title III); senior centers, (formerly provided under the old Title V); and nutrition services (previously addressed by the old Title

VII). A primary goal of these service systems is to maintain maximum independence of the elderly through the provision of support services with supplemental self-care.

State governments are allocated funds according to the number of persons aged 60 or older in the state as a proportion of all older Americans. Under the 1978 amendments, no state receives less than that received in fiscal year 1978. However, states will be required to increase their allocations to rural areas by 5 percent.

One state agency must be designated by each state to receive these funds and to develop and administer a state plan for the provision of services to the aging. The state agencies, in turn, must designate area agencies on aging (AAAs) to develop and administer local-area plans for "planning and service" areas. Area plans form the basis for the development of state plans, both of which must be prepared on a three-year basis, with annual adjustments as needed.

Local *planning and service areas* are flexibly defined; currently, an area can be any unit of general-purpose local government with a population of 100,000 or more. Other units of such size and areas adjacent may also be included to form a "regional planning and service area," when it can improve program administration. Area agencies may be any public or private nonprofit agency or organization, including an office of city or county government that has been appropriately designated for such planning.

Locally elected officials are to participate along with older individuals and the general public on advisory councils, established by each AAA to assist in planning. All the following social services may be funded under this title: health, continuing education, welfare, informational, recreational, homemaker, counseling, referral, services to access other social services including nutrition and housing, repair and renovation of housing, services to prevent institutionalization, legal services, financial counseling, preventive health, career counseling, state ombudsman, and services for the disabled. In addition, funding is available for altering, renovating, and, in some cases, acquiring facilities for use as multipurpose senior centers. Funds may also be used for assisting in the operation of such facilities, including outreach. A state ombudsman program, begun as a demonstration program under the act in the past, is now required in each state.

During fiscal years 1979 and 1980, to facilitate administrative consolidation of nutrition programs with other social service programs, areas may seek to use up to 20 percent of nutrition-service allotments for supportive services directly related to the delivery of congregate or home-delivered meals, including recreational activities, information and referral, and health and welfare counseling. (In such areas as Alaska, up to 50 percent can be used to allay unusually high costs.)

State allotments to AAAs are to be determined by a formula, reflecting the geographic distribution of individuals aged 60 and older. Each state is required to publicize the formula it develops for review and comment. Federal money may be used to pay for up to 75 percent of the AAAs' cost of administering area plans and up to 90 percent of the costs of services. In fiscal year 1981, the sharing of costs for services will shift from 90 percent federal and 10 percent state and local to 85 percent federal and 15 percent state and local, with the states responsible for bearing the whole cost of the 5 percent decrease in federal funds for these services. A maximum of 8.5 percent of Title-III funding may be used to cover expenses of administering area plans.

Each area is required to allot at least 50 percent of its social service dollars to three priority areas: access services (transportation, outreach, and information and referral); in-home services (homemaker/home-health aide, visting/telephone reassurance, and chore maintenance); and legal services. If these services are already sufficient to meet the need, this allocation may be reduced. Area plans are also to designate "where feasible" a focal point for the provision of these services. "Special consideration" should be given to the use of multipurpose senior centers for this purpose.

Title IV provides for the funding of evaluation, training, research, and demonstration efforts to be conducted by state and local governments and other public and private organizations, as follows:

1. Training programs for recruitment and for employment in programs for the aging. Under the 1978 amendments, special courses addressing the needs of rural providers are to be funded.

2. Research-and-development projects for determining elderly needs for service and for developing and evaluating new ways of addressing these needs such as problems in the delivery of transportation services, and the coordination of services by revising existing federal transportation programs for the elderly. Also addressed is the need to study comparative costs, problems, and needs for service delivery in urban and rural areas.

3. Demonstration projects to improve or expand social or nutrition services. Priority is given to funding of rural AAAs for addressing special needs of the rural elderly, including alternative health-care-delivery systems, advocacy, outreach, and transportation services. Special consideration is also given to projects that address special housing needs, including renovation and repair, and property-tax relief; needs for continuing education and preretirement education; needs of physically and mentally impaired older individuals for services such as special transportation and escort, homemaker, home health, and shopping; needs for alternatives to institutionalization through day-care and funding through state Title XIX and XX allocations; and needs of the rural elderly.

4. Demonstration projects in ten states will be established to coordinate social services for homebound elderly, blind, and disabled.

5. Comprehensive, coordinated long-term-care-system projects, for the development of systems emphasizing alternatives to institutionalization, assessment, care planning, and referral mechanism.

6. Legal-services demonstration projects to expand or improve the delivery of legal services to the elderly.

7. Model projects to relieve high utility and home-heating costs, with special consideration given to programs providing fuel or utility services to low-income elderly at reduced rates.

8. Multipurpose-senior-center-insurance revolving fund, providing insurance on mortgages (including advances on mortgages during acquisition, alteration, renovation, and construction). Mortgages that include the cost of equipment used in the operation of a new center are also to be insured. Annual interest grants may also be awarded for the acquisition, alteration, renovation, or construction of senior-center facilities.

9. Gerontology-center grants for establishing or supporting, in public and private nonprofit agencies, organizations for training, research, and program development, notably for long-term care and national-policy-study centers.

Title V (previously Title IX) authorizes the Department of Labor to provide grants to fund part-time community-service jobs for unemployed, low-income people (defined under the 1978 amendments as persons with incomes up to 125 percent of the poverty level) aged 55 years and older. Under this title, grants are available to two categories of contractors, states, and public and private nonprofit agencies and organizations. Preference in the second category is given to national organizations that have a "proven ability" in providing such services to older persons under similar programs. (Currently, eight national organizations have received grants, and are now providing 38,000 jobs, nationwide. States are providing 9,500 jobs nationwide.)

Jobs are extended to a greater number of individuals, and states are given larger roles in the program than previously. Spending authorizations for this title are $350 million for fiscal year 1979, $400 million for fiscal year 1980, and $450 million for fiscal year 1981. States are allocated 55 percent of the increase over fiscal year 1978 funding levels and national organizations or "contractors" 45 percent. Allocations within states may be evaluated for the distribution between rural and urban areas. To improve coordination between state agencies on aging and national contractors, all employment projects conducted under this title must be reported to the state office on aging thirty days before the project is undertaken for review and comment.

Provision is also made to assist workers in the transition to private employment. Traditionally, these community-service jobs have included: assisting policemen and social workers, repairing homes of the poor and elderly, assisting in senior centers, nursing homes, hospitals, schools, and many other public and private agencies. Technical assistance to help prime sponsors, businesses, and other organizations to create job opportunities through work sharing and other experimental methods is also provided for.

Title VI makes possible the development of social services, including nutritional services, for Indian tribes. Eligible tribal organizations must represent at least seventy-five individuals, aged 60 and older. Grants made under this title will cover all costs of service delivery.

The White House Conference of 1981 is authorized to develop recommendations for further research and action in the field of aging. Representatives of federal, state, and local governments, professionals, and citizens will be invited to participate.

The Domestic Volunteer Service Act of 1973 was amended, extending for three years the Retired Senior Volunteer Program (RSVP), Foster Grandparent Program, and Senior Companions and Health Aides (the "National Older Americans Volunteer Programs") which are operated under ACTION, the domestic equivalent of the Peace Corps Program and organized as a federal volunteer service agency. Elderly individuals with incomes up to 125 percent of the poverty level are eligible to be considered for the Foster Grandparent or Senior Companion programs.

The Age Discrimination Act has been strengthened with several new amendments. The provisions for enforcement now apply, with certain exceptions, to all age discrimination in programs using federal funds. Previously, this law was limited in its application to instances of "unreasonable" discrimination. In addition, these amendments provide individuals with the right to initiate action in claiming age discrimination, after administrative remedies have been exhausted.

Administratively, the act has also been strengthened, by giving HEW the authority to review and approve related regulations written by other federal agencies. All federal agencies will also be required to report to HEW on compliance with this law in all federally funded programs, including those administered locally.

The Commission on Civil Rights was to undertake a comprehensive study of discrimination based on race or ethnic background in federally funded programs affecting older individuals and to report its findings by March 1980.[25]

After a long delay the regulations to implement the Titles of the Older Americans Act Amendments of 1978 were issued in March 1980 and the stage was set to test the ramifications of these new provisions.

The Older Americans Act has resulted in the establishment of a nationwide network of agencies concerned with the elderly. At the federal level, the Administration on Aging, through regional offices, disburses the funds provided by the Older Americans Act and administers, monitors, and evaluates the programs of the various states. In turn, in each state there is a designated state unit on aging, which looks after the various community programs through a budgetary and planning review process. At the community level, area agencies on aging are designated that are responsible for the coordination of services and community resources.

In varying ways at the different levels of government, three basic strategies are engaged in the administration of the Older Americans Act; the first of these centers on the provision of services necessary to meet the objectives of the act. The Older Americans Act provides for services, and also it encourages the development of resources in other segments of government for the benefit of the elderly. A second strategy is the linking of people with services. This can include the provision of technical assistance by one agency to another to provide more effective services, the provision of information by an agency to an individual about available services and referring them to appropriate providers, and the location of individuals in the community unaware but in need of services. Finally, there is the strategy of advocacy in which agencies look after the rights and interests of the elderly population. This may take several forms, including developing legislation, monitoring programs administered by other governmental agencies to see that the elderly are receiving their proportionate share of the benefits, insuring that the rights of the elderly are not violated, and allowing the elderly full participation in the decision process that will influence their lives. The largest single source of other federal funding is from Title XX of the Social Security Act. These funds pay for the various social services that are within the jurisdiction of a state agency and also provide funds for training of personnel.

Other progrms benefiting the elders, paid for from social security funds and administered in other governmental agencies, include social security, SSI, medicare, and medicaid. Other federal programs that involve the elderly include the CETA (Comprehensive Employment and Training Act) and Senior Aides programs administered by the Department of Labor, VISTA, and RSVP in ACTION (see chapters 5 and 7). See Table 3-1 for an illustration of the level of funding in the budget presented by the Carter administration for the fiscal year 1981 in January 1980, prior to the revisions announced in March 1980 which contemplated a reduction by $40.3 million, or 6 percent below the January requests.

Differing Views and Issues

Caroll Estes in *The Aging Enterprise* takes a critical look at the underlying ideology of our national policies toward old people that the aged are special and different; that there is inevitability of physical decline; and that the

Table 3-1

Aging-Related Health and Welfare Programs, Federal Budget Proposal (1980)

(budget authority, in millions of dollars, by fiscal year)

Services	1979	1980	1981	Change/ 1980-1981
Office of Human Development Services				
State Agency on Aging	23.0	23.0	23.0	—
Social Services and Centers	197.0	247.0	280.0	+33.0
Nutrition	277.0	320.0	350.0	+30.0
Congregate Meals	(235.0)	(270.0)	(295.0)	(+25.0)
Home-Delivered Meals	(42.0)	(50.0)	(55.0)	(+5.0)
National Clearinghouse	2.0	2.0	2.0	—
Federal Council on Aging	0.45	0.45	0.58	+0.13
Training	17.0	17.0	17.0	—
Research	8.5	8.5	7.0	−1.5
Discretionary Programs/Projects	15.0	25.0	25.0	—
Long-Term-Care Demonstrations	(—)	(10.0)	(10.0)	(—)
Multidisciplinary Centers	3.8	3.8	3.8	—
Indian Tribes	—	6.0	6.0	—
White House Conference on Aging	—	3.0	3.0	—
Title 20 Basic Services	2,620.0	2,669.0	2,716.0	+47.0
Title 20 Training	90.0	89.0	116.0	+27.0
Health Care Financing Administration				
Medicare	29,148.0	33,542.0	37,349.0	+3,807.0
Medicaid	12,407.0	14,160.0	15,768.0	+1,608.0
Quality Assurance	29.0	30.0	34.0	+4.0
Research and Demonstration	16.0	24.0	28.0	+4.0
Long-Term-Care Demonstrations	(—)	(10.5)	(10.5)	(—)
Health Services Administration				
Community Health Centers	277.0	342.0	391.0	+49.0
National Health Service Corps	63.0	82.0	134.0	+52.0
Indian Health Service	492.0	549.0	602.0	+53.0
Hypertension	11.0	20.0	20.0	—
Home-Health Demonstrations	6.0	5.0	—	−5.0
National Institute on Aging				
Research	54.0	67.0	73.0	+6.0
Training	2.5	3.0	2.3	−0.7
National Institute of Mental Health	—	620.0	671.0	+51.0
National Institute on Alcohol Abuse and Alcoholism	175.0	190.0	201.0	+11.0
Social Security Administration (Outlays)				
Supplemental Security Income	5,471.0	6,374.0	6,925.0	+551.0
Energy Assistance	—	1,600.0	2,400.0	+800.0
Old-Age Survivors Insurance	90,129.0	104,029.0	121,163.0	+17,134.0

Source: Older Americans Report (February 1980).

problems of older people can be "cured" by services.[26] Since separatism and pluralism are the two major guidelines to our policies, setting the aged apart institutionalizes and legitimizes the marginality of the elderly, which, in turn, creates a network of providers in whose interests it is that the elderly continue to have needs that are met through services providers provide. In her view, the 1978 amendments reinforce existing power relationships between interest groups and focus attention on local power rather than on national objectives, emphasizing coordination when frequently there is nothing to coordinate, because essential programs simply do not exist. She points out that the major problem facing older people is social inequality and exclusion from the mainstream of American society and that the service strategy of the Older Americans Act is inappropriate to remedy this condition. On top, the fiscal resources allocated to the service programs under AOA and under Title XX of the Social Security Act are inadequate to do the job as outlined and promised. And decentralization engenders local-interest-group control rather than community control by the elderly to advance their well-being. Etzioni adds his view to support the same position:

in general older persons can be expected to benefit, in terms of their self-view and the image of them held by others, the more their problems are handled via broad-based "universalistic" social policies aimed at coping with social problems as they affect all citizens and the society at large, rather than via "particularistic" old-age-oriented policies, although these latter are necessary where more universalistic approaches are not available for one reason or another.

The view of older persons as a status group with unique specialized needs tends to set up a dysfunctional tension between older Americans and the rest of society. The tension is created by an implicit invoking or reinforcing of negative stereotypic images of older persons (in their own minds as well as in the minds of others). They tend to type them as victims of social segregation, physical isolation, and discriminatory attitudes and perhaps also serve to incur resentment toward them as a social albatross that must be borne by the rest of society.

This tension would be much reduced if more general, societywide policies replaced categorical programs in taking care of older persons' special needs. Needless to say, such policies are also more likely to have wide and lasting public support than policies which seek to benefit a subgroup, however sizable, powerful, and well organized.[27]

The debate on the merits of the universalist versus the particularist approach is likely to become more vocal and may enter into the deliberations of the White House Conference of 1981. In addition, the holistic versus segmented approach will come in for scrutiny, as contained in this question: What attempts are being made to view the needs or problems of the elderly holistic and inseparable from one another, rather than to view them piecemeal with attendant piecemeal solutions that further segment the program and service structure and demand new mechanisms to achieve coordination of the segmented parts?

Joseph A. Califano, Jr., former secretary of HEW, in an address before the Select Education Subcommittee of the Committee on Education and Labor (U.S. Senate) in March 1978 made the following statement:

> We believe that this Conference (in 1981) will provide a similar forum to that in 1971; a forum for developing comprehensive approaches to the problems that will confront the Nation's elderly citizens over the next generation.
>
> Some difficult and deeply serious problems confront us: Over the past two decades, Federal, State and local agencies have rapidly expanded these programs to serve older people. But our compassion has too often exceeded our understanding. We have created a virtual maze which is often incomprehensible to the older people we are supposed to serve. Now we must take the time to re-examine carefully the organization and delivery of our services if they are to meet the pressing needs of the next decade.

The following questions are relevant and need to be addressed by the delegates of the 1981 conference:

1. How can we ensure that the support systems respond effectively to the widely varying circumstances of the elderly and their families?

2. How can we make certain that the efforts of government actually enhance and add to the compassionate care and support of families for their elders? (In some cases, government interventions may strain rather than strengthen family life.[28])

3. How can we halt the fragmentation, waste, and duplication that have come with proliferation of programs for the elderly at every level of government? Today officials and elderly alike in thousands of communities call for a drastic reduction of paper work and for simplification of rules and regulations that erect barriers for the elderly rather than open up opportunities for them.

4. How can we build a partnership with state and local governments to improve the management and delivery of services to the frail elderly and the chronically impaired to secure and maintain maximum independence and dignity in a homelike environment for older individuals capable of self-care with appropriate supportive services? How can we remove individual and social barriers to economic and personal independence for all older individuals and provide necessary services to the more vulnerable minority elderly?

5. How can we build incentives into the system of care that will encourage the least restrictive care in each case, and how can we insure and protect the right of elderly citizens to choose their own alternatives?

6. By what criteria and mechanism will an individual's needs be evaluated and measured or a provider's services be rated?

7. How can we be sure that the entrance of a public program into a community does not cause the exit of other programs—especially volunteer efforts. Or, stated differently, how can voluntary efforts of the informal (natural) network be harnessed and combined with the formal, bureaucratic service structure to the benefit of all parties concerned?

In the next four chapters we will take a look at the major needs areas of our aging population and various major programs that have been designed, developed, and implemented, either in accord with evolving social policies or on an ad hoc basis to respond to political forces, economic imperatives, value orientations, or sheer opportunism. The needs areas to be discussed are by no means inclusive or all encompassing. Those needs areas were selected that constitute the major social-policy priorities in any society, because they address existential needs that, in the Maslow scheme, are basic underpinnings for the satisfaction of higher needs of a population: income, health, housing, and social supports.

Notes

1. "Social-Cultural Contexts of Aging: Implications for Social Policy," Andrus Gerontology Center, University of Southern California, Los Angeles, California, 1976.

2. Robert Morris, *Social Policy of the American Welfare State* (New York: Harper and Row, 1979), p. 17.

3. Florence Kluckhohn, *Personality in Nature, Society, and Culture* (New York: Alfred A. Knopf, 1953), p. 21.

4. M. Borges and L. Dutton, "Attitudes toward Aging: Increasing Optimism Found with Age," *Gerontologist* 16 (April 1976):236-242.

5. H. Rosencrantz and I. McNevin, "A Factor Analysis of Attitudes toward the Aged," *Gerontologist* 9 (November 1971):55-59.

6. Robert W. Kubey, "Television and Aging: Past, Present and Future," *Gerontologist* 20 (February 1980):16-35.

7. Robert Butler, *Why Survive? Growing Old in America* (New York: Harper and Row, 1975), p. 12.

8. Vern Bengtson, *The Social Psychology of Aging* (New York: Bobbs-Merrill, 1973).

9. Elaine Cumming and Henry William, *Growing Old—The Process of Disengagement* (New York: Basic Books, 1961).

10. Gordon Streib and C.J. Schneider, *Retirement in American Society* (Ithaca, N.Y.: Cornell University Press, 1971).

11. Robert Binstock and R. Hudson, "Political Systems and Aging," in

R.H. Binstock and E. Shanas, eds., *Handbook of Aging and the Social Sciences* (New York: Van Nostrand Reinhold, 1976).

12. *Facts about Older Americans*, U.S. Department of HEW Administration on Aging, DHEW Publ. no. (OHDS) 79-20006, 1978.

13. Francis Carp, "Impact of Improved Housing on Morale and Life Satisfaction," *Gerontologist* 15 (June 1975):511-515.

14. G. Gutman and C. Herbert, "Morality Rates among Relocated Extended Care Patients," *Journal of Gerontology* 31 (1976):352-357.

15. White House Conference on Aging, "Toward a National Policy on Aging," vol. 1, "Background, Organization, Program," 1971, p. 10.

16. Ibid.

17. Ibid., vol. 2.

18. Robert Binstock, "Aging and the Future of American Politics," *The Annals of the American Academy of Political Science* 415 (1974):199-212.

19. David H. Fisher, "The Politics of Aging in America, A Short History," *The Journal of the Institute of Socio-Economic Studies* 2 (1979):51-66.

20. Robert Hudson, "The Graying at the Federal Budget & Its Consequences for Old Age Policy," *Gerontologist* 18 (October 1978):428. Reprinted by permission of *The Gerontologist*, 1835 K Street, N.W., Suite 305, Washington, D.C. 20006.

21. Louis Lowy, *Social Work with the Aging: The Challenge and Promise of the Later Years* (New York: Harper and Row, 1979), pp. 194-195.

22. Robert Binstock, "Aging and the Future of American Politics," *The Annals of the American Academy of Political Science* 415, 199.

23. Hudson, "Graying at the Budget," p. 435.

24. *Older Americans Act of 1965, As Amended*, Administration on Aging, DHEW Publication, July 1979.

25. U.S., Congress, House, *Older Americans Act: A Summary*, Staff Study, Select Committee on Aging, August 1978.

26. Carroll L. Estes, *The Aging Enterprise* (San Francisco: Jossey-Bass, 1979), chap. 1, pp. 1-15.

27. Amitai Etzioni, "Old People and Public Policy," *Social Policy* (Nov./Dec. 1976):21. © 1976 by Social Policy Corporation. Reprinted with permission.

28. Marjorie H. Cantor and M.J. Mayer, "Factors in Differential Utilization of Urban Elderly," *Journal of Gerontological Social Work* 1 (1978):49-50, 59.

4 Income Policy and Programs

Economic support of an older population is not only a fiscal but also a political question. To what extent is our society willing to redistribute its economic resources to make it possible for older people to live in dignity and reasonable comfort? The combination of three societal trends, the demographic, economic, and employment, can seriously threaten both the elderly's income security and the financial viability of the government support programs. Although the present income program structure has reduced poverty among the elderly, poverty, as we have seen in chapter 3, is still disproportionately high. Moreover, the present economic structure makes it unlikely that during the later years of life an aged person will be able to maintain a standard of living equivalent to that enjoyed earlier in life. Although it is true that persons retiring today are relatively better off than their predecessors, retirement, even at age 70, for many persons still significantly increases the probability of severe income loss, decline in living standard, and downright impoverishment. And that probability increases the longer inflation continues at high rates. This development occurs against the backdrop of a dawning recognition on the part of public policy makers that the financing of the Social Security Act must be rethought.

A recent study concluded that: "After more than a decade of expanded government interest and support, the elderly nonetheless find themselves losing ground; year by year their economic position has grown worse."[1] This steady deterioration in the elderly's economic well-being is attributable to the inflation the nation has been experiencing—an inflation the magnitude and character of which have changed dramatically. The "creeping" inflation (2 to 3 percent per year) of the 1960s has become the "galloping" inflation (10 to 15 percent and higher per year) of the 1970s. Moreover inflation has come to be characterized by a "hard-core" base, which persists even during periods of high unemployment and is clearly distinguishable from the cyclical, demand-pull type that tends to appear as full employment is approached. Finally, and most importantly from the elderly's viewpont, the market-basket items that have come to register the highest annual rates of price increase are necessities such as food, housing, fuel, and medical care—items that consume a far higher share of the budget of the elderly family unit than of the nonelderly. One only need examine the inflation figures that are now available for 1980: not only did the aggregate rate total 15 plus percent, but the rates for necessaries, especially food and medical care, were at even higher levels. And let it be understood, our present income policy toward the aged is basically one of assuring a minimum standard of income adequacy rather than one of income maintenance.

The Elderly's Income

A 1977 Congresional Budget Office (CBO) study isolated the impact of government programs on the incidence of poverty. The study showed that, were it not for income from social-insurance programs, 59.9 percent of all families headed by an elderly person would have fallen below the subsistence-based poverty line in fiscal 1976. Social-insurance programs, dominated by social security, reduced that elderly poverty rate from 59.9 percent to 21 percent. Cash-assistance programs, such as supplemental-security income (SSI) reduced the rate even further to 14.1 percent.

In-kind benefit programs, like medicare and food stamps, also made a contribution. According to the CBO study, when the value of these benefits is cashed out and included in income, the percentage of elderly in poverty in fiscal 1976 was reduced to 6.1 percent. Although calculating the impact of in-kind benefits on income status yields interesting findings, the CBO data should not be accepted as a new measure of poverty, especially when comparing poverty rates among age groups. Of all the benefits in the CBO's in-kind category, medicare and medicaid benefits contribute the most "income" to the elderly (the sicker you are the richer you are).[2]

One of every nine couples with a husband 65 or older received incomes less than $4,000 in 1976. At the other end of the income scale, one of every five elderly couples had incomes of $15,000 or more. The median income for thes couples was $8,070. The income of elderly persons living alone or with nonrelatives was more skewed to the lower end of the income distribution. Nearly two of every five received incomes under $3,000, and only one of five received more than $6,000. The median income for these individuals was $3,495 (see figure 4-1).[3] Major sources of income for older people include: earnings from salaries, wages, and self-employment; property ownership; social security (social-insurance) benefits; supplemental-security income; public assistance (general relief); veterans, unemployment, workmen's compensation; and retirement income (private or public pensions). (Table 4-1 and figure 4-2 provide a statistical overview.)

Social Security Program

Social security benefits are the single most important source of income for the largest number of older people in all industrial societies. Everywhere

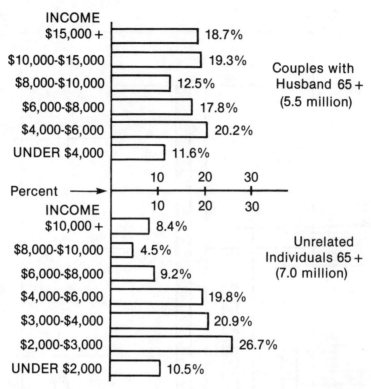

INCOME
$15,000 + 18.7%
$10,000-$15,000 19.3%
$8,000-$10,000 12.5%
$6,000-$8,000 17.8%
$4,000-$6,000 20.2%
UNDER $4,000 11.6%

Couples with
Husband 65 +
(5.5 million)

Percent ⟶   10   20   30

INCOME
$10,000 + 8.4%
$8,000-$10,000 4.5%
$6,000-$8,000 9.2%
$4,000-$6,000 19.8%
$3,000-$4,000 20.9%
$2,000-$3,000 26.7%
UNDER $2,000 10.5%

Unrelated
Individuals 65 +
(7.0 million)

Source: U.S. Department of Health, Education and Welfare, Office of Human Development Services, *Facts about Older Americans*, DHEW Publication (OHDS) 79-20006 (Washington, D.C., 1978).

Note: For couples, data are restricted to 2-person families in order to exclude income received by other family members in larger families.

Figure 4-1. Persons 65 and Older: Percent Distribution by Income (1976)

such income is strictly transfer. It is earned by the younger workers but is allocated to the elderly no longer at work. And the young provide for the old in the expectation that they will be provided in turn.

Originally established in 1935 under the Social Security Act (Title II), the major income program of social insurance is financed through compulsory contributions from employers, employees, and the self-employed. The program initially offered only retirement benefits for industrial and commercial workers, but was subsequently expanded to include disability insurance and benefits for the survivors and dependents of the insured workers. Coverage has been extended to include most of the following: self-employed persons, state and local government employees, employees of charitable, educational, and religious organizations, members of the armed

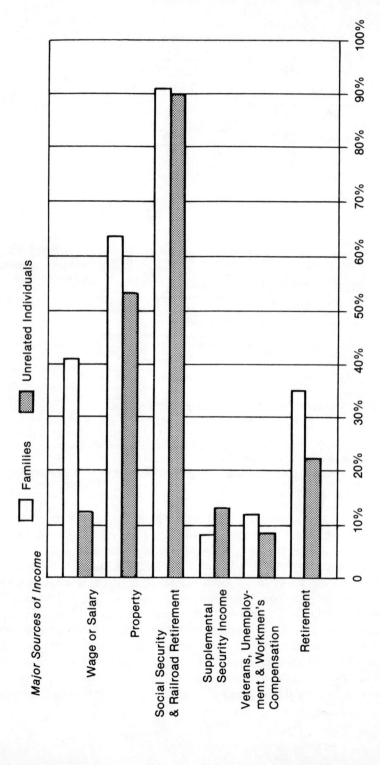

Source: U.S. Bureau of the Census, *Current Population Reports*, unpublished data.

Figure 4-2. Distribution of Major Income Sources among Families and Individuals Aged 65 and Older (1975)

Table 4-1
Percentage Receiving Income from Different Sources among Families and Individuals Aged 65 and Older (1975)

	Families	Unrelated Individuals
Earnings		
Wage or salary income	41.7	13.5
Nonfarm, self-employment income	7.5	2.4
Farm self-employment income	5.9	2.1
Income Other than Earnings		
Property income, total[a]	64.4	53.8
Social security and railroad retirement income	90.9	90.1
Supplemental-security income	8.4	13.9
Public assistance or welfare	2.7	2.1
Veterans, unemployment, and workmen's-compensation income	12.3	8.6
Retirement income, total[b]	35.7	22.9
Other income, total[c]	2.9	2.2
No Income	0.1	0.8
Selected Combinations of Income Sources		
Earnings	49.6	17.5
Earnings and property income	3.3	1.5
Government transfer payments	94.5	95.1
Public assistance, SSI, or both	3.8	15.1
Social security, retirement income, or both	92.8	92.1
Social security, SSI, or both	92.1	92.5

Source: Unpublished U.S. Bureau of the Census data.
[a]Interest, dividends, net rent, estates or trusts.
[b]Private pensions, annuities, military-retirement pensions, federal-employee pensions.
[c]Alimony or child support, regular contributions, other.

forces, household employees, and farm workers. Today, nine out of ten workers are earning social security coverage; nearly one out of every seven American citizens receives monthly social security benefits. The social security program touches almost every American family in some way.[4]

Although other programs, including medicare, medicaid, and supplemental-security income, have been established under the Social Security Act, the term *social security* popularly refers only to the Old Age, Survivors and Disability Insurance program (OASDI). The following description includes only the OASDI program, which is administered entirely by the federal government through the Social Security Admnistration (SSA) and its approximately 1,300 branch offices. (Descriptions of medicare and medicaid are in chapter 5 on health policy.)

Eligibility

Whether one is eligible for social security retirement benefits depends not on need but on earnings from what the Social Security Administration calls *covered employment* or *self-employment*. Almost all jobs are included in covered employment, but some jobs in government, a few with charitable, religious, and educational institutions, and some family and domestic employment are not covered. About 90 percent of jobs are in covered employment, and for these jobs the law requires that social security taxes be reported by the employer.

Length of time in covered employment from 1950 to 1 January 1978 is counted by calendar quarters, a three-month period beginning January 1, April 1, July 1, and October 1 of each year. If a person has had 40 quarters of coverage at any time, he or she is fully insured for life. Otherwise, to be fully insured a person must have at least 1 quarter of coverage for every year after 1950, but not including the year he or she reaches age 62. The quarters may have been earned at any time—before or after 1950 or before or after age 21—as long as the total number is sufficient.

No matter how much workers earn, they cannot obtain more than 4 quarters of coverage in a single calendar year. A self-employed individual generally obtains 4 quarters of coverage if his or her self-employment income for a calendar year is $400 or more and none if it is less than that. There are, however, special rules that permit agricultural workers to obtain quarters of coverge on a more liberal basis.

Work Credit for Retirement Benefits

Year Worker Reaches Age 62	Number of Quarters Needed for Benefits
1975	24
1976	25
1977	26
1978	27
1979	28
1983	32
1987	36
1991 or later	40

(There is a special provision for persons who became 72 before 1970 and did not have enough quarters of coverage for regular benefits. Depending on the year the person became 72, it is possible to qualify without any quarters of coverage or with a reduced number.) Fully insured workers are eligible for retirement benefits for the month in which they reach age 62 or age 65.

Full benefits are available at age 65. If retired workers elect for their benefits to commence between ages 62 and 65, the monthly payments are permanently reduced.

A person need not be fully retired to receive benefits. Retirees aged 62 to 72 can earn as much as $5,000 a year in 1980 without receiving any deductions from their benefits. This amount is referred to as the *retirement test* or *earnings limitation*. It is subject to go up every year as the cost of living rises. (The exempt amounts are expected to be $5,500 in 1981 and $6,000 in 1982.) However, income from securities, savings accounts, rents, and pensions do not count toward the earnings limitation. The age at which the retirement test no longer applies will be lowered from 72 to 70 in 1982. Since 1978, the earnings limitation are applied annually to everyone so that persons making the same amount of money during the entire year will receive the same level of benefits. The monthly measure will be retained, however, during the first year of retirement to allow those who retire in the middle of the year to collect benefits during the months when they are not working.

Family members of a retired worker may also be eligible for benefits that are called *auxiliary benefits*. The wife of a retired worker, even though she has never been in covered employment, is eligible for benefits in her own right when she reaches the age of 62 (reduced benefits) or 65 (full benefits). She need not be living with her husband. If she is under 62, she can still receive benefits if she is caring for an under-18 child of the retired worker or a disabled child of the worker. The divorced wife of a worker can collect benefits if she is not currently married and was married to the retired worker for at least ten years.

The wife's benefit is generally 50 percent of that paid to the retired insured worker. If the wife is eligible for benefits from her own work record, she cannot collect the wife's benefits in addition—she can only collect the larger of the two benefits. This is the case with other persons who seem to meet the requirement for two different types of monthly benefits. They cannot receive both, only the larger of the two.

The husband of a retired worker can collect benefits based on his wife's earnings record when he attains the age of 62 (reduced benefits) or 65 (full benefits) and can demonstrate that more than one-half of his support was furnished by his wife. A husband can now collect benefits if he is under 62 and is caring for his wife's minor child. In 1977, however, the Supreme Court decided that it was unfair to require widowers to prove dependency to receive benefits when widows did not have to do so. Because of the recognition that the present laws are sexist and inequitable, the Social Security Administration is now studying ways to bring about equal treatment of men and women throughout the system and to submit proposals to Congress for changes.

Benefits can be paid to each dependent child of a retired worker if the child is unmarried and under 18 (or under 22 if a full-time student) or is disabled and became disabled before 22. Benefits are one-half the amount paid to the retired parent, subject to a ceiling on total family payments. Illegitimate children are included under certain circumstances.

Amounts of Benefits

The amount of the monthly social security check is based on the past earnings of the retiree. (The exact computation of benefits requires precise information about the worker's past earnings and the use of formulas and charts available at a social security office or in Social Security Administration publications.) Generally, however, a worker's average monthly wage is computed for the years since 1950, or for those born after January 1, 1930 for the years after they reached age 21. The worker is allowed to drop out years of lowest earnings. Then the average monthly wage is converted to the primary insurance amount, which represents the maximum monthly benefit available to the retired worker.

There is a ceiling on the amount of earnings creditable to social security so that beyond a certain point, a worker's earnings cannot increase the social security benefits. The ceiling figure (or taxable wage base) has been steadily upgraded throughout the last twenty-five years. From 1951 to 1954 the maximum amount was $3600, in 1976 the maximum was $15,300, and for 1980 it is $122,200.

The maximum monthly benefit payable to a retired worker generally would be over $400. The minimum retirement benefit for a worker retiring at 65 will be frozen at the minimum level in effect in January 1979 (about $121).

The amount of the monthly benefit does not remain frozen. Congress can legislate across-the-board increases in benefits as it sees fit. As of 1972 there is a provision for an automatic benefit escalator whenever the cost of living increases by 3 percent or more and Congress has not taken action to increase benefits.

The entire amount of social security benefits goes to the retiree; social security benefits presently are not subject to federal income taxes. (Several policy analysts and politicians have proposed that a proportion be subject to taxation to bolster the funding reservoir of social security.)

Survivor's Insurance

The survivor's-insurance component of social security provides cash benefits to family members of an insured worker who dies.

Eligibility. Generally, for survivor's benefits, the deceased person must have met the same fully insured test applicable to retirement benefits. A worker born after 1 January 1930, however, is fully insured if he or she had 1 quarter of coverage for each calendar year elapsing after the year he or she attained age 21 and before the year of death or disability. Also, if there are surviving dependent children, there is a currently insured category with a less stringent eligibility standard. To have been currently insured when he or she died, the worker need have had only 6 quarters of coverage during the 13-quarter period before his or her death.

If the deceased husband met the eligibility standards, his widow is entitled to receive benefits at age 60 (or 65 for full benefits). If the widow is disabled, she can begin to receive benefits at age 50. A surviving divorced wife who had been married to the deceased worker for at least ten years is similarly entitled to benefits. If the widow remarries after age 60, she can still continue to receive benefits. If the widow remarries before age 60 or if a surviving divorced wife remarries at any age, she will not be entitled to benefits until the subsequent marriage ends.

A widow or surviving divorced wife is entitled to benefits (called "mother's benefits") regardless of her age if she is caring for a child of the deceased worker. If the mother remarries, eligibility for benefits ceases for the duration of the subsequent marriage.

A surviving dependent child is entitled to child's insurance benefits if he or she is under 18, or under 22 and a full-time student, or has a disability that commenced before age 22.

A widower of an eligible deceased wife is entitled to widower's benefits if he is over 60 (or over 50 and disabled). A 1977 Supreme Court decision held that it was unfair for widowers to have to prove that they received over one-half of their support from their wives when widows did not have to prove that their husbands had supported them. The Social Security Administration is now studying ways to bring about equal treatment of men and women throughout the system. A widower over the age of 60 who remarries will not have his benefit reduced.

A dependent parent of the deceased worker can also receive benefits if he or she is over 62 and received at least one-half his or her support from the deceased worker.

Amount of Benefits. Generally, widows, widowers, and surviving divorced wives are entitled to the same amount that would have been paid to the worker if he or she had retired. Children and mothers under 60 are entitled to 75 percent of this amount. Dependent parents are entitled to 82.5 percent (or 75 percent each if both parents are surviving) subject to reduction if they become entitled before age 65. The amount of benefits can be reduced if the recipient remarries or works and earns more than the annual exempt amount. There is also a maximum family benefit, which limits total family benefits to roughly 1.5 times the amount that would have been paid to the worker if he had retired.

In addition to regular survivor's benefits, a special lump sum death payment of $255 is made to the widow or widower of the deceased worker. To be eligible, the surviving spouse must have been living in the same household with the deceased at the time of death. If there is no eligible widow or widower, the payment goes to the person who paid for the burial expenses of the deceased worker (or to his estate if it paid).[5]

Disability Insurance

Originally added to the Social Security Act in the 1956 amendments, the disability-benefits component assists those workers under age 65 who are unable to perform any substantial gainful work. When a disabled beneficiary reaches age 65 the payments are converted to retirement benefits. To qualify, a worker must meet medical and employabillity criteria for disability as well as insured-status requirements for social security coverage. A worker is fully insured if he or she has 40 quarters of coverage or, if less, 1 quarter of coverage for each year after 1950 (or after the year he or she attained age 21, if born after 1 January 1930) until the year before he became disabled. Those receiving disability payments may also be eligible for SSI payments, and they are eligible for medicare after two years as a disability beneficiary. Family members of a disabled worker are entitled to auxiliary benefits similar to those of family members of a retired worker.

Disability. As defined by the Social Security Act *disability* means an inability to work caused by: (1) any severe physical or mental impairment that has lasted or is expected to last at least twelve months or to result in death; or (2) blindness.

In Social Security Administration regulations, there is a "Listing of Impairments"—certain serious impairments and illnesses that automatically qualify a worker for disability, unless he or she is in fact performing substantial work. Examples of such disability conditions include: blindness, loss of two limbs, certain severe hearing losses, various advanced diseases of other body systems, and severe mental disorders. The claimant has the burden of producing medical evidence to prove that his condition falls within one of the listed impairments. Even if the worker does not have a listed impairment, the claimant will be eligible if he or she has a "medically determinable" impairment, or combination of impairments, equally severe to those listed.

If disabled workers do not have a listed impairment or its equivalent, they may still prove that their medical condition prevents them from engaging in substantial gainful activity. This can be a difficult standard to meet. Substantial gainful activity means not just the claimant's previous line of work but any reasonable work "which exists in the national economy." Thus, it does not matter if they cannot perform any work that exists in their immediate area or if they cannot be hired because of shortage of work or discrimination against the disabled. However, the claimant's age, education, and work experience will be taken into consideration.

If claimants earn more than $200 per month at any kind of work, they are presumed to be able to engage in substantial gainful activity. However, individuals 55 or older who meet the statutory test of blindness may earn more than this if they are in a different line of work than they engaged in before they became blind.

If a worker has been found eligible for another disability program such as workmen's compensation or veteran's disability, this does not establish disability for Social Security. It is quite possible to meet the disability standards of another agency yet be not disabled for social security purposes. And vice versa, if workers are barred from workmen's compensation, for example, they may still be eligible for social security disability benefits.

Eligibility. As with retirement and survivor's benefits, the worker needs to have built up a sufficient amount of work credits to be eligible for disability payments. The number of quarters of coverage necessary depends on the age of the worker when disabled. In addition to being fully insured those age 31 or older who do not meet the test of blindness must have at least 20 quarters of coverage out of the last 40 and a younger person must have coverage for at least half the quarters that elapsed after age 21, and, in any case, at least 6 quarters.

When workers become disabled, a "disability freeze" is put on their earnings records to protect their own or their family's eventual entitlement to retirement or survivor's benefits. Thus, the entire period of disability—a time of low or no earnings—will not be considered when the worker's insured status and level of benefits are determined for retirement or survivor's insurance, and his period of disability will not count against him in computing required quarters of coverage.

A worker can receive workmen's compensation and still be fully eligible for social security disability benefits. However, if the combined total monthly payments to the worker and his family exceed 80 percent of the worker's average monthly earnings before the disability, the social security benefits will be reduced.

Auxiliary Benefits. The same family members who are entitled to benefits from a retired worker's coverage are also entitled to auxiliary disability benefits. These include: wife over 62; dependent husband over 62; wife (any age) caring for a child under 18; unmarried children under 18 (or under 22 and full-time students); or children who became disabled before age 22 and continue to be disabled.

Termination of Benefits. If the worker's medical condition improves to the extent that he or she is no longer disabled, benefits are still payable for a two-month adjustment period following the month in which the disability ceases. If the worker is still disabled but seeks to return to work (perhaps under a state rehabilitation plan), there is a trial work period of nine months during which benefits continue, regardless of the amount of earnings. If the worker finds that he or she is able to work successfully beyond the nine-month period, he or she can still receive two additional months of adjustment payments until benefits cease. Disability benefits are also terminated on the worker's death or when the worker attains age 65, at which time benefits are automatically converted to retirement benefits at the same payment level.

Amount of Payments. The amount of the monthly payment does not depend on the extent of the disability but on the worker's average earnings as under other social security programs. The range of benefits that could be paid to a single disabled worker is from $107.90 to about $600. The maximum family payment for the highest creditable level of earnings is about $875.[6]

Supplemental Security Income

In 1974 the major welfare program for the aged, blind, and disabled, "Old Age Assistance" (OAA), was replaced by the "Supplemental Security Income" (SSI) program under Title XVI of the Social Security Act. It was hoped that the program would result in poor people having more cash to spend; a national minimum income for the aged, blind, and disabled; uniform eligibility conditions instead of conditions that differed widely from state to state under OAA; a start in unraveling the administrative snarl enveloping welfare programs (SSI is federally administered by the Social Security Administration).[7]

There are two types of benefits under SSI: the basic federal payment and optional state supplementary payments. However, legislation passed in 1973 obligated states to supplement the federal payment to at least maintain 1973 state OAA levels (in cases where these 1973 levels were higher than the 1974 federal minimum income). The maximum federal SSI benefits for an individual and a couple without other income and living in their own household were $1,752 and $2,628 in 1974. As a federal cash-benefit program for the aged, blind, and disabled, it guarantees basic, uniform income levels to needy aged, blind, and disabled persons in all fifty states and the District of Columbia.

SSI is administered primarily by the Social Security Administration through its district offices. SSI, however, is entirely distinct and separate from the OASDI component of Social Security, the major difference being that eligibility for SSI is based on need, whereas OASDI is based on an individual's past work and earning level.

Eligibility

To be eligible for SSI, a person must meet four basic requirements: (1) One must be either aged (65 or over), blind, or disabled. (2) One must have an income below a certain specified amount. (3) One must possess resources— total property other than income—less than a certain amount. (4) One must meet certain general qualifications such as U.S. residency and U.S. citizenship (or resident-alien status).

Categorical Definitions

To qualify as aged, persons must establish that they are 65 years or older, and the technical definition of blindness states that one's vision with best correction be 20/200 or less in both eyes or that one have a visual field restricted to 20 degrees or less. The definition of disability under SSI is the same as that under the disability-insurance program of Social Security. As in the case of disability for social security insurance purposes, the actual disability determinations are made by state agencies, not the SSA office.

A person who received aid to the blind under a federally aided state program in December 1973 and met the blindness test in effect for that program as in effect in October 1972 will be considered blind so long as she or he continues to meet that definition. A person who received Aid for the Disabled under a federally aided state program for December 1973 and at least one month prior to July 1973 on the basis of a disability definition in effect in October 1972 shall be considered disabled so long as he or she continues to meet that definition.

Limited-Income Requirement

To be eligible for SSI, an applicant must have less than a certain level of *countable income.* As of 1977, the income levels were $177.80 monthly for an individual or $266.70 for a couple. These figures are raised each June as benefits change because of cost-of-living increases. In determining the income level, all the applicant's income is considered—whether earned or unearned, whether in cash or services. Then, certain exclusions are applied to reach countable income. Countable income is also the key to determining how much the applicant will get once he is found eligible.

Earned income includes gross wages earned in employment and earnings from self-employment; unearned income includes all income other than wages and self-employment earnings such as pensions, retirement payments, workmen's-compensation payments, and Social Security benefits; support and maintenance furnished in cash or in-kind; alimony payments; proceeds of a life-insurance policy in excess of $1,500; dividends and interest; and inheritance.

Deemed income is another form of unearned income. When an eligible adult lives with an ineligible spouse, part of the income of that spouse is "deemed" to be available as income to the SSI applicant. The idea behind deeming of income is that persons living together as a family unit have an obligation to each other to share resources. (Of course, if both spouses are eligible, they are considered as a couple, with higher income permitted and higher benefit payments.)

Once the applicant's total income has been computed, certain exclusions or deductions can be applied. The most important of these are: (1) a $60 per quarter exclusion that can be applied to any income except for benefits based on need; and (2) the first $195 per quarter plus one-half the remainder of earned income. Irregularly received income of up to $30 per quarter (earned) or $60 per quarter (unearned) can also be excluded. (This included gifts and income from occasional work.)

An Illustration

Mr. Almond receives $105 a month in wages and $80 a month as workman's compensation. His wife, who is ineligible for SSI, receives $200 a month in earnings.

Mr. Almond		*Mrs. Almond*	
$125	monthly wages	$180	monthly wages
− 65	earned-income exclusion (1/3 of $195 quarterly exclusion)	− 65	work-expenses deduction (1/3 of $195 quarterly)
60	total	115	total

Mr. Almond   *Mrs. Almond*

− 30	(1/2 of remainder)		− 84	wife's allocation (1/3 of $252)
30	countable earned income		$ 31	deemed income to husbands
+ 80	unearned income			
110				
− 20	general-income exclusion			
	(1/3 of $60 quarterly exclusion)			
90				
+ 45	deemed income			
$135	countable income (The monthly amount otherwise payable will be reduced by the amount of countable income.)			

Resource Limitations

Resources are essentially all things of value owned by an individual, including cash assets, one's home, and personal property. The SSI limitation on resources, after exclusions, is $1,500 for an individual and $2,250 for a couple. All the resources of a spouse are deemed to be available to the other spouse and must be applied toward the resource-limitation ceiling. In some cases, state resource limitations under prior welfare programs were more liberal than the current SSI standard. In most instances, a person who was regularly receiving state aid in December 1973 and before can continue to use the state resource test.

Includable Resources. All liquid resources are counted without exclusion toward the resource limitation. Liquid resources are those that can be readily converted into cash, including bank accounts, stocks, bonds, and some trusts. Nonliquid resources include all real property and personal property not readily convertible into cash. There are numerous exclusions for nonliquid resources, so that it may be worthwhile for an applicant to convert liquid into excludable nonliquid assets so as to meet the resource limitation.

Excludable Resources. Some of the major resource exclusions and their limits are:

Resource	*Resource Limit*
Home	No limit on value
Household goods and personal effects	$1,500; wedding ring and engagement ring and needed medical devices are totally excluded

Resource	Resource Limit
Automobile	
General use	$1,200 retail value
Used for job transportation	Totally excluded
Used to obtain regular medical treatment	Totally excluded
Specially equipped for disabled person	Totally excluded
Insurance	
Term life insurance	Totally excluded
Other life insurance	Up to $1,500 face value
Burial insurance	Totally excluded
Property used for self-support (that is, business or other income-producing property)	Excluded in reasonable amount

Excess Resources. If the applicant has countable resources in excess of $1,500 or $2,250, it may be worthwhile to dispose of or convert the excess resources. There are three ways to carry this out:

1. The person can change countable resources into excludable resources. For example, one could excess cash to buy a home, automobile, or household goods within the limit.

2. One can transfer excess resources, by gift or sale. The transfer must be legally binding and not revocable or otherwise a sham transaction.

3. In certain instances, the person can agree to dispose of excess resources and in the meantime receive conditional SSI benefits. Then, after the sale of the property, the balance of the proceeds in excess of the resource limitation must be applied toward paying back the conditional SSI benefits.

Such transactions are quite painful for people; they still are in accord with the pauper philosophy of the English Elizabethan Poor Laws.

Other Eligibility Considerations

There are several additional eligibility requirements besides the age, disability, and financial tests.

Residency and Citizenship. The SSI recipient must be a resident of the United States and either a U.S. citizen or an alien legally residing in the United States.

Institutionalization. If SSI applicants are full-time, that is, for more than one month "inmates of a public institution," they may be eligible only for greatly reduced SSI benefits or none at all. The notion behind this is that if the person's basic needs are being met, full SSI payments are not necessary.

If a person is in a public or private institution, such as a hospital or nursing home, and medicaid funds pay more than 50 percent of the cost of care, he or she is eligible only for a $25 maximum monthly benefit. Thus such an individual would receive $25 less any countable income. if the applicant is in a public facility not receiving medicaid funds—such as a prison—he or she is not eligible for any benefits.

Other Available Benefits. The SSI applicant is required to apply for all other benefits to which he or she might be entitled. These would include pensions, retirement benefits, veteran's benefits, and so forth. The SSA has the responsibility to determine whether there is probably eligibility for other benefits for which the person must apply.

Rehabilitation. Blind and disabled applicants may be required to accept state vocational rehabilitation services as a condition of eligibility. Also, claimants who are disabled partly because of alcoholism or drug addiction are required to accept available treatment for their condition.

Amount of Benefits and Income

Presently, the maximum monthly benefit available to an SSI recipient is $177.80 ($266.70 for a couple). However, one's actual payment may be less, depending on income and living arrangement. The countable-income figure used in computing one's eligibility for SSI is also used in computing the SSI payment. This "countable income" is simply subtracted from the $177.80 or $266.70 payment maximum to arrive at the monthly benefit.

Living Arrangement

If an SSI claimant is not living in his own home, his benefits can be affected. As has been already noted, residents of public institutions may have their benefits eliminated or greatly diminished.

The other important situation is when the SSI recipient is "living in the household of another," which means receiving support and maintenance (room, board, and incidentals) in another person's private home. If the recipient is in this category, his benefit standard of $177.80 (or $266.70 if a couple) is automatically reduced by one-third.

If the recipient is making a payment for his room and board, he must be able to prove that the payment is similar to what it would cost to rent an apartment and buy his own food.

If the claimant is receiving only board or only room, the reduction does not apply, but the value of the room or board must be computed and treated as income. And the reduction does not apply if, although not owning the home, the claimant can show that he or she is equally sharing in all the costs of the household.

Typical Benefit Standards (as of June 1977)

	Monthly	Quarterly
Eligible individual	$177.80	$533.40
Eligible couple	266.70	800.10
Individual in institution	25.00	75.00
Couple in institution	50.00	150.00
Individual in household of another	118.54	355.62
Couple in household of another	177.87	533.40

Two Illustrations

Jane Mitchell is elderly, lives alone, and has a part-time job at which she earns $220 per month. Her SSI benefit payment is calculated as follows:

Countable Income	*SSI Benefit Payment*
$660 gross quarterly earned income	$533.40 quarterly benefit std.
− 60 general-income exclusion	− 202.50 countable income
600	
− 195 earned-income exclusion =	$330.90 quarterly benefit
($195 + 1/2 the remainder)	
405	
− 202.50	Monthly SSI benefit is $110.30
$202.50 countable income	($330.90 divided by 3)

Paul Robins is 70 years old, collects a pension (not based on need) of $60 a month ($180 a quarter), and lives in the home of a friend. Mr. Robins contributes only a nominal sum toward his room and board and does not share equally in the household expenses.

Countable Income		*SSI Benefit Payment*	
$180	quarterly pension (unearned)	$533.40	quarterly benefit std.
− 60	general-income exclusion	− 177.80	1/3 reduction for living in another's household
$120	countable income	255.60	
		− 120.00	countable income
		$235.60	quarterly benefit payment

Monthly SSI benefit is $78.53 ($235.60 divided by 3)

Representative Payees

The SSA can designate a third party—called the "representative payee"—to receive checks for the SSI claimant when the SSA determines that this course is in the best interests of the claimant.

If the claimant is an alcoholic or a drug addict, a representative payee must be appointed. Otherwise, the SSA has wide discretion to decide if a representative payee is advisable. The only applicable standard is whether the recipient has the capacity to manage his or her payments and protect his or her interests.

Usually, a close relative is appointed as the payee or, if there is none, a friend or the social agency or institution responsible for the individual's care. The representative payee can only use the funds for the claimant's basic needs and is required to submit periodic reports to the SSA accounting for the expenditures.

There are two forms of state supplementation of SSI benefits. One is a mandatory state supplementation for those who were receiving greater benefits under the prior state program. The other is an optional supplementary payment offered by those states that wish to augment SSI benefits. Supplementary benefits are available in almost three-fourths of the states.

Mandatory State Supplementation. Each state must put up any funds needed to maintain the former level of benefits to certain aged, blind, and disabled recipients who received aid under its federally assisted state program in December 1973. This process of protecting most of the recipients who were transferred from a state to the federal program is called "grandfathering." State recipients grandfathered into the federal SSI program may have the benefit of: (1) less strict definitions of blindness and disability (as previously described); (2) higher resource limitations; (3) additional amounts for essential persons; and (4) for the blind only, a higher amount of income disregarded.

Optional State Supplementation. Although it is not required by the federal law establishing SSI, states that offered higher benefits under their state plans may continue to offer those higher payments to persons newly qualifying for SSI. The amount of this optional supplementation varies greatly from state to state and also varies according to the recipient's condition (aged, blind, or disabled), marital status, and living situation (whether in his own home, institutional care facility, and so forth).

As of February 1977, forty-one states and the District of Columbia offered some form of optional supplemental payments to, for example, an aged individual living independently. The supplements can be administered through a separate payment by the state or can be paid by the state to the federal government, which includes in it the payment to the recipient. At present twenty-five states administer their own optional supplementation, and sixteen states and the District of Columbia have the federal government administer it.

Posteligibility Considerations

Redeterminations and Reporting Requirements. The Social Security Administration conducts periodic (usually annual) redeterminations of SSI recipients' eligibility, generally by a personal interview. In addition, the recipient has an obligaton to report any changes in circumstance that might affect eligibility. Some of the specific events that must be reported are: change in address or living arrangements; change in income; change in resources; eligibility for other benefits; change in marital status; admission to or discharge from a hospital or nursing facility. Failure to report these events promptly may result in the imposition of a penalty.

Suspensions and Terminations. SSI benefits will be suspended or terminated when the recipient no longer meets the eligibility requirements. Termination is a permanent cessation of benefits that occurs when: (1) the recipient's blindness or disability ceases; (2) the recipient's benefits have been suspended for twelve months as for income or resources above eligibility limits; and, of course, (3) the recipient dies.

Suspension is a temporary cessation of benefits that occurs when the recipient fails to meet eligiblity requirements, but termination does not apply. The most common reasons for suspension are: (1) excess income; (2) excess resources; and (3) becoming an inmate of a public institution (other than one in which medicaid pays for more than half the care). As soon as the recipient again meets the eligibility requirements, his benefits will be reinstated.[8]

SSI, although federally administered, is still subjecting individuals to means testing and therefore retains a welfare stigma. For this reason, many older persons are reluctant to subject themselves to what many conceive of as degrading interrogations by SSI officials to bar their assets and to qualify for so-called charity handouts. One cannot say that the SSI program is designed to enhance a person's sense of self-worth and dignity. In fact, the Poor Law philosophy inherent in the program fosters a punitive attitude and creates a demeaning climate of welfarism that further alienates the elderly poor from the mainstream of self-respecting nonpoor, old and young.

Private Pensions

From 1960 to 1970, private-pension-plan coverage increased from 21.2 million to 30 million workers. During this same period, assets of these private plans increased from $52 billion to $138 billion. At the present time, the value of assets held is well in excess of $250 billion, with a growth rate of about $20 billion a year.

Generally, a *pension* can be defined as any fund, plan, or program that provides retirement income to employees or results in a deferral of income by employees until the termination of employment or beyond.

There are two basic types of penson plans. In the defined or fixed-benefit plan, the employer promises that the employee will receive a fixed benefit (pension) on retirement in terms of dollar amount or on a per-centage basis. For example, the plan may say that the retiring employee will receive 50 percent of final average pay. In the defined-contribution or purchase-money plan, the employer promises to put in a fixed amount each year that will be allocated among employees based on their age, length of employment, and rate of pay. On retirement, a pension annuity will be pur-chased from insurance companies with the money invested in the account of the retiring employee.[9]

In a profit-sharing plan, the company lets employees participate in a share of the employer's profits; they are considered to be pension plans under the Employee Retirement Income Security Act of 1974 (ERISA), the law that now governs the creation and administration of private pension plans. The act's purpose is to protect the interests of workers and their beneficiaries who depend on benefits from employee pension plans. The law requires disclosure of plan provisions and financial information and establishes standards of conduct for trustees and administrators of welfare and pension plans. It also sets up funding, participation, and vesting requirements for pension plans and makes termination insurance available for most pension plans. The act preempts all state laws that relate to employee benefits plans subject to ERISA, even if there is no conflict between the state law provisions and ERISA. The law does not require all companies or unions to establish private pension plans for their employees or members. In fact, half the private work force is not covered by pension plans. Most of the provisions of ERISA to protect workers do not apply to people who stopped working before 1976. ERISA does require that existing or new plans meet certain minimum standards.

The law is administered primarily by the Department of Labor and the Internal Revenue Service. In addition, the pension-plan-termination insurance program is administered by a corporation established within the U.S. Department of Labor—the Pension Benefit Guaranty Corporation.

Coverage

The act covers employee pension and welfare plans that are established or maintained (1) by an employer engaged in commerce or any industry or activity affecting commerce, or (2) by any employee organization or organizations representing employees engaged in commerce or industry or activity affecting commerce, or (3) by both, except those plans specifically exempted. Because of the broad interpretation of the language "affecting commerce," the vast majority of private pension plans should be presumed to be under the mandate of the act.

The act specifically exempts several types of pension plans from its coverage. Included in this group of excluded plans are governmental plans; certain church plans that do not elect coverage; plans maintained solely to comply with workers' compensation, unemployment compensation, or disability-insurance laws; non-United States plans covering nonresident aliens; and so-called excess-benefit plans (plans that provide benefits or contributions in excess of those allowable for tax-qualified plans that are unfunded—that is, no monies are specifically set aside for later payment of pension benefits.

Standards

The act imposes a federal "prudent man" rule on fiduciaries (individuals entrusted with pension-plan monies or responsible for the administration of the plan) in the management of private pension plans. Administrators must file various reports with the Department of Labor, the Pension Benefit

Guaranty Corporation, and the Internal Revenue Service. These reports include descriptions of the plan, the EBS-1 form, and the annual report, ordinarily form 5500.

Employers are also required to file with the Social Security Administration information on an employee's vested pension benefit when he or she leaves a job. The SSA will then provide this information to participants and beneficiaries on request and also on their application for social security benefits. This requirement should provide a valuable record of benefits earned to retirees and should provide in the future a critical source for social workers attempting to find "lost" benefits previously earned by older people.

Age and Service Requirements

Workers who are participants in a pension plan generally receive credit toward a pension for those years they worked for an employer contributing to the plan. Participation alone, however, does not mean that a worker has a right to receive a pension. This depends on the plan's vesting provisions.

Generally, a pension plan must allow an employee to participate when he or she is age 25 and has completed one year of service. There are exceptions. Any plan providing full and immediate vesting may require an employee to put in three years of service before he or she is eligible to participate. Also employees covered under a collective-bargaining agreement may be excluded for purposes of the coverage requirements if there is evidence that pensions have been the subject of good-faith bargaining. An employee can be required to put in a year of service before being covered by a pension plan. The amount of time necessary to qualify for participation may vary from industry to industry. Once minimum-age and service requirements are met, participation must begin at the start of the next plan year or six months after meeting the requirements, whichever is earlier.

A plan may not exclude an employee because she or he is old. The act does permit defined-benefit plans (those plans that guarantee a retiring employee a final sum of income) to exclude an employee who is within five years of normal retirement age. The reason for this exclusion is to avoid discouraging a company that maintains a defined-benefit plan from hiring older employees because of the cost of funding benefits for them. A plan may provide that no benefits are to be paid to a participant until the tenth anniversary of the date when he or she began work. Thus a participant whose period of employment began late in his or her career may not be eligible to receive plan benefits until some time after reaching normal retirement age.

The law says a break in service occurs in any year in which an employee has no more than five hundred hours of service. The Labor Department is considering an alternative method for calculating both years of service and breaks in service. If an employee returns to his job after a break in service, certain rules apply. Generally, all service under the plan with the employer is to be taken into account for participation. However, the plan may require a one-year waiting period before aggregating prebreak and postbreak service. After the effective date of ERISA in 1976, the only way a worker could lose previous pension credits is if he were not vested when he had a break in service and his period of absence equalled or exceeded his years of service before the break. For example, if an employee works for three years, quits without being vested, and then returns to employment after a break of three years or more, the plan need not give him credit for the initial three-year period.

Vesting

When employees become eligible for participation in a pension plan, they will receive credits toward their pension for all years they worked for an employer contributing to a plan—with some important exceptions. After an employee has worked a specified period of time for an employer contributing to a pension plan, the act requires that he or she be given the right to receive certain benefits on retirement—even though he or she leaves that job before retirement. This right is called *vesting*.

Under certain circumstances, a worker can get vesting credit for years worked during which he was not a plan participant. These nonparticipating years need not be counted for benefit-accrual purposes (years counted in determining the dollar amount of a pension).

A pension plan covered by vesting provisions must provide full and immediate vesting of benefits derived from employee contributions. Employer contributions must vest at least as fast as provided under one of the following schedules: (1) full (100 percent) vesting after ten years of service (with no vesting prior to completion of ten years of service); (2) graded vesting (five to fifteen years)—25 percent vesting after five years of service, plus 5 percent for each additional year of service up to ten years (50 percent vesting after ten years), plus an additional 10 percent for each year thereafter (100 percent vesting after fifteen years of service); and (3) rule of 45 (based on age and service)—50 percent vesting for an employee with at least five years of service when his age and years of service add up to forty-five, plus 10 percent for each year thereafter. Under any of the options an employee must be at least 50 percent vested after ten years of service and 100 percent vested after fifteen years of service. In addition, the law provides that a person will be vested if he is participating and working at normal retirement age, even though he has less than ten years of service.

The vesting requirements did not take effect, in most cases, until after 31 December 1975. When they did go into effect, however, the requirements took into account all a worker's years of service with the employer. There are exceptions. Years of service before the plan was subject to the vesting provisions need not be counted if such service would have been disregarded under the plan's rules on break in service in effect on the applicable date. Service before 1971 must be recognized only if the employee earned credit for work in at least three years. An employee may also lose vesting credits if he has a break in service that equals or exceeds his years of service before the break.

A plan may provide for the forfeiture of the employee's vested benefits derived from employer contributions in the event of the employee's death before retirement. A plan may provide for suspension of a retiree's benefit payments for the period of his reemployment if a retiree returns to work for his employer, or, in the case of a multiemployer plan, during the period a retiree is employed in the same industry and trade or craft and in the same geographical area covered by the plan.

Benefits

The amount of benefits paid on retirement depends on the number of years of participation. There must be at least two continuous years of participation, however, to qualify for a pension. Benefit-accrual credit may also be lost for breaks in service before vesting that equal or exceed the years of service before the break.

Rules governing when benefit payments begin have the dual purpose of guaranteeing that pension-plan benefits will primarily be used as retirement income and providing that the pension plan will have sufficient time to fund the benefit payments. Under the act, payments begin when the latest of the following events occurs: (1) the individual attains age 65 or earlier normal retirement age; (2) the tenth anniversary of the time when the participant begins service; or (3) the participant employee terminates his service with the employer.

When the act was written, the sponsors recognized that one reason widows and to an increasing extent widowers are a severely disadvantaged economic group was because the death of the retired employee often caused a total loss of pension income to the surviving spouse.

The act attempts to remedy this occurrence in several ways. Under the act, where a retirement plan provides that a participant may take his benefits in the form of an annuity, as most pension plans do, it must also provide for a joint and survivor annuity, provided the participant has been married for one year prior to death and one year before the annuity starting date and does not elect in writing to give up the survivor annuity. A joint and survivor annuity provides periodic payments of money to the surviving spouse after the original annuitant (in this case the retired employee) dies.

The annuity payments to the survivor must not be less than one-half the annuity payable to the participant while he and his spouse are both living. As a result of this survivor-annuity requirement, the benefit payable to the employee may be reduced to reflect the additional actuarial cost of the survivor's benefit.

Some pension plans provide for early retirement. ERISA states that if a plan provides for early retirement and an employee continues to work without taking early retirement, the plan must provide him or her with an opportunity to convert what otherwise would have been his early-retirement benefit into a joint and survivor annuity that will be payable to his surviving spouse if he dies while working for the employer.

Even with the improvements in widow-widower protection brought about by the act, there are some problems. Even if the employee makes the early-retirement election, the survivor will still not receive benefits if the employee dies of natural causes within two years of making the election. Also, if the worker dies before early-retirement age, the survivor gets nothing. Finally, in plans that do not provide for early retirement, the survivor will not get any benefits if the worker dies before retirement age.

Legislation has been proposed to improve the situation; section 205 of ERISA would be amended to require private pension plans to provide a survivor's annuity for the spouse of an employee who dies before reaching retirement age equal to the survivor's annuity to which the spouse would have been entitled if the employee would have retired the day before his death.

Many private pension plans are integrated with the social security payment program. Nevertheless, ERISA prohibits reductions in private-pension-benefit payments to a retiree because of an increase in social security benefits or wage base once a retiree has started receiving pension benefits.

Portability

When employees leave a pension plan in which they have vested benefits to take a new job, these vested benefits are transferred to the pension plan of the new employer. The act initiates the first step toward establishing uniform portability procedures. It calls for voluntary agreements between employers to transfer vested benefits between plans. For such transfer to occur, three parties would have to agree—the old employer, the employee, and the new employer.

Critics of this portion of the act say that the first step is really no step at all because no incentives are given the old employer to give up control of the pension-fund money. Without this agreement, of course, no transfer is possible.

Protection of Pension Benefits

One of the goals of the pension-reform movement was to guarantee that pension benefits earned by employees would be available when the employee retired. The act insures up to a maximum amount benefits of participants in covered defined-benefit pension plans. A defined-benefit pension plan is one that promises a future benefit that is stated in the plan or can be calculated according to a formula stated in the plan.

There are important limitations on the insurance coverage. Possibly the most important is that only vested-employee benefits are insured under the plan. In most cases an employee will have to work ten years before benefits are protected from business failure, merger, or the like. Several kinds of plans are not included under the insurance-coverage provisions. Two of the most important categories are plans exempt from the law's coverage: governmental plans, church plans, and so on, and plans that do not provide for employer contributions (such as union-dues plans).

There are many possible civil actions that may be brought under the act. For example, participants and beneficiaries may bring an action to enforce their rights under a pension plan and to recover benefits due to them. They may also bring an action to clarify their rights to future benefits. Injunctive relief (a court order to refrain from doing a particular act) is available against any act or practice that violates any reporting, disclosure, participation, vesting, funding, or fiduciary provision of the act, or the terms of their plan. Employees may also bring suit if they are fired, or disciplined to deprive them of pension rights.

Generally, a civil action under ERISA must be filed in the federal courts. A suit based on breach of contract can be filed in a state court, but it is subject to transfer to the federal courts by either party if an interpretation of the act is involved.

Congress, by enacting ERISA, has begun an extended program of private-pension reform. The act does much to guarantee protection of employee rights and benefits under private pension plans. However, ERISA is only the first milepost. For that reason, it is important to reiterate what the act does not do. The act does not require employers to offer pension plans to employees. If an employer should establish a plan, then the act requires that the plan meet certain minimum standards. The Congress also placed no provision in the act dealing with adequacy of pension benefits, and in some instances the law provides that surviving spouses may receive nothing at all. Termination insurance does not cover all pension plans; it covers only defined-benefit plans that meet other specified standards and only those that terminate after 1 July 1974. Finally, and most importantly, the act, with few exceptions, does not provide help to those retirees who have lost rights or benefits prior to 1976.

The Senate Labor and Human Resources Committee in 1980 took a look at yet another piece of legislation to simplify ERISA, aimed at reducing or eliminating the volumes of paperwork associated with the program.

The ERISA Simplification Act carries five provisions, four of which slash paperwork requirements. The fifth proposal in the bill would give the Treasury Department power to enforce ERISA rules through civil actions. Pursuit of cases is currently handled by the Labor Department.[10]

Public Pensions

Federal, state, and local employee pension-plan programs are rapidly growing sources of retirement income for older people. These programs often provide benefits to both covered employees and their survivors. Unlike private pensions, there is no single law that provides guidelines for the creation and maintenance of public retirement systems. Two applicable federal laws are the Civil Service Retirement Law and the Railroad Retirement Act.

Each public retirement program is administered by its own particular federal, state, or local agency. For example, the civil service retirement system is administered by the Civil Service Commission, and the railroad retirement pension plan is administered by the Railroad Retirement Board. At present, there are no uniform requirements to guide the management and operation of public treatment programs.[11]

Problems with Pensions

A major segment of the work force still remains uncovered. It is difficult to make private pensions inflation-proof; very few private pensions adjust for general price increases during retirement; the economic costs of private-pension administration, investment, mobility, disclosure to recipients, and regulation are much higher than for social insurance. It is difficult to make private pensions portable—that is, to allow workers to have job mobility without a reduction in the value of their pension rights relative to what the value would be if they did not change jobs; private pensions may discourage the hiring of older workers because it is usually more costly to provide such workers with a specified pension benefit; and private pensions contribute to the concentration of corporate ownership and control.[12]

Schulz et al. recommend adoption of an adequacy-of-income standard for social security old-age benefits, which would provide inflation-protected benefits equal to at least 55 percent of the individual's or family's (if married) preretirement average earnings during the best of ten of the last fifteen years prior to retirement. The balance of retirement income would come from private pensions and savings.[13]

Other Sources of Income

Employment, noncash incomes, and tax benefits are other main sources for older people to meet some of their financial and economic needs, although they do not provide for income security on a universal basis.

Employment

In 1977, about 2.9 million or 13 percent of older people were in the labor force—either working or actively seeking work; they make up 3 percent of the U.S. labor force. One-fifth of the older men (1.8 million) and about 8 percent of the older women (1.1 million) are in the labor force. However, about 5.1 percent of older people in the labor force were unemployed. The balance (2.8 million) were employed. One-sixth of older men who work are in agricultural jobs, and over one-third are self-employed. The male labor-force-participation rate has decreased steadily from two of three older men in 1900 to one in five in 1977; the female rate rose slightly from one in twelve in 1900 to one in ten during the 1950s, but it dropped to one in twelve in the 1970s (see figure 4-3).[14]

In light of the demographic, economic, and elderly labor-force-activity trends, it would make good sense for the government to permit and encourage greater labor-force participation on the part of older persons and for older persons to take advantage of the employment incentives and opportunities created. Increased elderly employment activity would generate additional tax revenue for use at all levels of government. The economy in general would benefit from the added production of goods and services and from improved productivity levels. The elderly would benefit by being able to supplement their income from other sources with income from employment, thus increasing their ability to maintain, if indeed not enhance, their standard of living and do it with a form of income (wages) that has better prospects for keeping up with inflation than other forms of income. Finally, any share of that income that can be generated through the work effort of willing and able elderly individuals represents a share that need not be borne by other workers through taxes.[15]

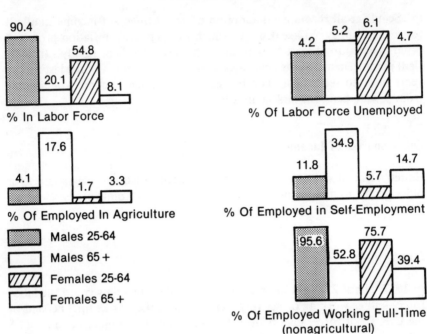

Source: U.S. Department of Health, Education and Welfare, Office of Human Development Services, *Facts about Older Americans*, DHEW Publication (OHDS) 79-20006 (Washington, D.C., 1978).

Note: Charts drawn at different scales.

Figure 4-3. Work Experience (1977)

A national, coordinated older-worker-employment strategy should be directed to the elimination of existing elderly-employment barriers, the greatest of which are the legal sanctions that permit discrimination. Unlike the fair-employment laws that protect all women and members of racial minorities, the fair-employment statutes protect only some older citizens and prohibit only some discriminatory practices.

In 1978, Congress enacted amendments to the Age Discrimination in Employment Act (ADEA) that prohibit mandatory retirement before age 70, with a few exceptions, and protect most federal employees completely against age-based retirement. These amendments do not go far enough. The repeal of statutory sanctions for forced retirement and of the statutory exclusion of persons over 70 from the enjoyment of the rights created by the act is a major goal. Legally sanctioned forced retirement must end if the expansion of employment opportunities and the creation of work incentives aimed at older persons are to be successful in reversing the downward trend in elderly employment.

The second major objective of an older-worker-employment strategy should be the elimination of existing work disincentives. The chief disincentive—the social security earnings test—serves to discourage (or in some cases bar) work effort by older persons. Another disincentive is age-based discriminatory employment practices, which continue to exist despite the protection of the ADEA. Added to that is the fact that the ADEA itself sanctions some of these practices.

The third objective of an older-worker-employment strategy should be the creation of new or the modification and/or expansion of existing government employment programs aimed at elderly workers. At present, the federal policy response is limited to two program—the Senior Community Services Employment Program (SCSEP), funded under the Older Americans Act, and the Comprehensive Employment and Training Act (CETA) Program.

The SCSEP is the only categorical program focused exclusively on older workers. It provides a small number (fifty thousand) of part-time jobs for workers age 55 and over who have been chronically unemployed and are below the poverty level at program entry. This program has developed into a manpower program, emphasizing on-the-job training with the objective of placing trained workers in permanent, unsubsidized jobs.

It is clear that barriers and economic disincentives that drive or discourage older workers out of the labor market must be eliminated and that work incentives (like actuarially increased social security benefits for those who elect not to apply for them until after age 65) and special employment programs aimed at older workers must be created or expanded. It is also clear, however, due to the widespread misconception concerning the so-called uniformity of productivity declines among older people, that these actions will still not be enough to maximize elderly labor-force participation. Changes on the demand side (the employer side) will also be required.

Employers need to be given incentives to employ and/or retain older workers. The federal tax structures ought to be used to provide such incentives (and at the same time provide incentives to older workers to take advantage of the work opportunities so offered). For example, the employer portion of the social security payroll tax that would otherwise have to be paid with respect to older workers could be reduced or eliminated. A tax credit for a certain portion of the older worker's income could also be used to encourage employers to hire them.

Food Stamps

The Food Stamp Act of 1964 affirmed a congressional commitment to the goal of providing adequate levels of nutrition for all segments of American society. The act and its amendments established the Food Stamp Program to supplement the purchasing power of low-income households that meet certain criteria established by the Department of Agriculture. Using these national standards based on family size and income level, state and local welfare agencies process applications and certify eligibility.

Food stamps are not free. Households pay a certain sum based on their family size and income level and receive food stamps of a larger value than the amount paid. The purchase requirement was eliminated by an amendment in 1978 to the Food Stamp Act. These stamps can be spent like money in authorized stores to buy almost any foods, or seeds and plants to grow food. However, they cannot be used to buy liquor, beer, cigarettes, soap, or other nonfood items. The elderly who are disabled or housebound can use food stamps to pay for home-delivered meals-on-wheels and for group meals for the elderly.

As of 1979 food stamps can be "cashed out"—that is, people can receive money in lieu of food stamps. A survey by the U.S. Department of Agriculture Food and Nutrition Service in 1975 revealed that 27 percent of all households surveyed were headed by persons 66 and over consisting of one or two persons. The low, fixed incomes of many older persons often make supplementary sources of income for the purchase of food a necessity. In addition, older persons pay a disproportionate share of their budget for basic items such as food and shelter. Inflation compounds these problems.

Eligibility. Food stamps are given to two kinds of households: public-assistance households and non-public-assistance households. Public-assistance households are ones in which every person in the household gets some form of state or federal welfare; they are automatically eligible for food stamps. A non-public-assistance household is one in which either some people get welfare and others do not or no one gets welfare. Non-public-assistance households are eligible for food stamps if they meet certain income and resources tests. Persons receiving SSI are automatically eligible for food stamps, unless they live in California or Massachusetts, if: (1) they live alone or with other SSI recipients; or (2) they live with a public-assistance household; or (3) they live with others but as a separate household.

A *household* is a group of people (except roomers and boarders), whether related or not, that meets three requirements. The group must share common cooking facilities; the group must usually buy food together; the group must live together as an economic unit. One person living alone is a one-person household.

Income and Resources Requirements. Most SSI recipients and all public-assistance households are automatically eligible for food stamps. But non-public-assistance households must meet income and resources tests. Generally, income is money received on a regular basis (such as wages, public assistance, retirement, disability benefits, pensions, veterans, or workman's or unemployment compensation, social security benefits, strike benefits, alimony, dividends, interest, and so on). A resource is other money or property. Resources include liquid assets such as cash on hand or in a bank or other savings institution; U.S. Savings Bonds; stocks and bonds; and such nonliquid assets as buildings (except for the family home and lot), land, and certain other real or personal property. Besides meeting these income and resources criteria, certain household members must register for and accept suitable employment.[16]

Tax Benefits

In addition to property-tax relief, several state governments grant to the elderly other types of tax relief, including exemption of prescription drugs from sales tax and certain income-tax breaks—special income levels for filing returns; higher personal exemptions; special medical deductions; special treatment of retirement income; and tax credits. Additional federal tax benefits to the elderly through income-tax laws include:

A double personal exemption: persons age 65 or older can deduct from their taxable income an additional personal exemption, which in 1980 is equal to $1000

Exemption from taxation of benefits received under the social security and railroad retirement systems: social security benefits are excluded from gross income as are railroad retirement benefits

Retirement-income credit intended to extend tax benefits (somewhat comparable to the tax benefits resulting from the exclusion of social security and railroad retirement from gross income) to retired individuals who are not covered (or only partially covered) by the social security and railroad retirement programs

Sale-of-personal-residence-capital-gains exclusion: persons who sell their home on or after their fifty-fifth birthday and who owned and used it as their principal residence need not include in their income any gain on the sale.[17]

Table 4-2 presents an overview of federal benefits as they have changed from 1971 to 1978.

Table 4-2
Federal Benefits for the Aged, by Type of Benefit (1971 to 1978)

Type of Benefit	Benefits (bil. dol.)								Percent		
	1971	1972	1973	1974	1975	1976	1977	1978	1971	1975	1978
Cash benefits	34.2	38.1	46.0	53.2	64.7	73.0	72.2	76.9	77.7	79.6	74.0
Social security	27.1	30.2	37.1	42.8	51.8	58.6	56.6	62.9	61.6	63.7	60.6
Railroad employees	1.7	1.9	2.1	2.3	2.8	3.2	5.6	3.0	3.9	3.4	2.9
Federal civilian employees	2.3	2.7	3.3	4.3	5.5	6.4	4.4	5.0	5.2	6.8	4.8
Military retirement	0.7	1.0	0.7	0.8	1.1	1.2	1.8	2.0	1.6	1.4	1.9
Coal-miners' widows	0.1	0.1	0.2	0.2	0.2	0.2	0.3	0.3	0.2	0.2	0.3
Supplemental-security income[a]	1.4	2.2	1.1	1.4	1.8	1.8	1.7	1.9	3.2	2.2	1.8
Veterans pensions	0.9	—[b]	1.4	1.4	1.5	1.6	1.8	1.8	2.0	1.8	1.8
In-kind benefits	9.8	10.5	11.0	12.5	16.6	19.0	22.9	27.0	22.3	20.4	26.0
Medicare	7.5	8.4	9.0	9.9	12.8	15.0	18.3	21.5	17.0	15.7	20.7
Medicaid	1.9	1.7	1.5	2.2	2.6	3.0	3.3	3.8	4.3	3.2	3.7
Food stamps	0.2	0.2	0.1	0.1	1.0	0.6	0.8	0.5	0.5	1.2	0.5
Subsidized public housing	0.2	0.2	0.3	0.2	0.4	0.4	0.5	1.1	0.5	0.6	1.1
Total outlays	44.0	48.6	56.9	65.7	81.3	92.0	95.1	103.9	100.0	100.0	100.0

Source: U.S. Office of Management and Budget, *The Budget of the United States Government*, annual.

Note: For years ending June 30, except beginning 1977, ending September 30.

[a] Prior to 1974, represents federal grants to states for aid to the aged, blind, and disabled.

[b] Veterans pensions included in supplemental-security income.

Major Issues and Options

One of the major policy issues in relation to the economic security of older persons has to do with measures to assess the economic standard and to test the adequacy of the programs. The two most widely used measures for aged families are SSA's poverty and low-income indexes and the U.S. Bureau of Labor Statistics' "Budget for a Retired Couple." These indexes have been useful for setting levels of income above which minimum income adequacy is indicated. But the levels established by these indexes are arbitrary—being based in the case of the social security index on an emergency food budget and the assumption that these food costs constitute one-third of total required living expenditures. In the case of the Bureau of Labor Statistics' budgets, the designated levels are above a minimal level and seek to provide something called a "modest but adequate" living standard.

Viewing the adequacy of retirement income in terms of preretirement-earnings replacement is becoming more common in developing pension policy.[18] The standard used, however, is oriented toward maintaining the existing socioeconomic class structure—and liberal proponents would argue for a review of the minimum-level principle and urge that an income guarantee—commensurate with prevailing economic standards—be provided to all elderly.

Another issue relates to the continued financing of the social security program. Payroll deductions of equal shares by employees and employers are regressive because the proportion the contribution represents of total earnings falls for earning levels above the maximum-taxable-earnings ceiling. As benefit levels are increased, these contributions become an increasingly burdensome and inequitable tax on the poor worker. Congress has used the social security system as a welfare system for the aged (minimum benefits, weighted-benefit formulas, and early eligibility) but has not financed these welfare benefits with general-revenue financing. As the population "ages" with a rising percentage of the population age 65 or older, rising pension costs are projected to exceed payroll-tax contributions.

Some options presently being discussed by Congress to put the social security program on a sounder fiscal footing include: Financing aged health care insurance (medicare) out of general revenue and using the released funds for old-age pension financing; removing the 7 percent limitation on the tax rate for the self-employed and raising the tax to 150 percent of the employee contribution rate; and raising the age of eligibility for social security retirement benefits. Greater benefit reductions for those who retire before age 65, and an increased benefit for those who delay work stoppage until after age 65, with the added attraction of icreasing the amount of earnings a person can have before benefits are reduced, would help the program considerably. Also eliminating work disincentives and having more older people in the labor force will go a long way toward alleviating some of the financing problems currently projected for the Social Security system, as will elimination of the ceiling of the amount taxed through payroll deductions; use of general revenues for the entire program; elimination of the retirement test; and taxing part of benefits earned.[19]

The experiences of other countries (over 130 countries have some type of social security program) will provide valuable data for study and experimentation here. Although there is wide variation from country to country, some generalizations can be made. Slightly more than half of pension programs work under social-insurance tripartite financing (employee, employer, and government contributions); in most countries old-age benefits become payable between ages 60 and 65, although in some countries the age is as low as age 50 and in a few it is as high as age 70. Over half of the programs have the same pensionable age for women as for men, the others permit women to retire earlier; a majority of programs impose a retirement test in determining benefit eligibility, although some industrial countries have already eliminated it, notably West Germany and treat social security benefits as an annuity. Pensions in most countries are wage-related, but computation methods vary greatly. The majority of programs add supplements to pensions if a recipient has a wife or young children. Most countries provide survivor's benefits that typically is a fixed percentage of the prior pension.[20]

A third major issue relates to the elimination of SSI as a stigmatized welfare program. An option would be to incorporate it into the federal insurance program and maintain a special social-assistance program to meet crises, emergencies, special contingencies, or catastrophic events that may befall older people on a case-by-case basis.

The fate of private and public pensions will be of continuous concern by Congress, as witnessed by further legislative proposals to insure vestedness, portability, and inflation buffers. Also, tax-relief measures can be a major source of income provision for those elderly who qualify by virtue of their more advantageous economic position in the social structure. Options would include: use of preferential tax rates for widows and widowers; an automatically increasing measure of tax relief to be targeted for those elderly-income components that are relatively fixed, such as private pension benefits and interest from savings accounts; and elimination of double taxation of dividend income.

In the final analysis the income conditions of older persons are related to the economic conditions of the country. Economic growth, inflation, unemployment, allocation of the economic pie based on societal values, support for competing economic claims, and moves toward reducing inequality for the total population are the powerful variables that affect any income policy for the elderly. In other words, the economic well-being of older persons is intimately linked to the economic well-being of all people in any society. And poverty of the young and the old can be eliminated if a society makes it one of its main social priorities and designs an antipoverty strategy to accomplish this goal primarily with economic and income measures available to all industrialized nations rather than relying primarily on a service strategy.

Notes

1. U.S., Congress, Senate, *Developments in Aging*, part I, A Report of the Special Committee on Aging, 1978, 95th Cong., 2d sess., chap. 2, pp. 31-41.

2. *U.S. Congressional Budget*, U.S. Government Document Publication (Washington, D.C.: U.S. Government Printing Office, 1977).

3. U.S Department of Health, Education and Welfare, Office of Human Development Services, *Facts about Older Americans*, DHEW Publication (OHDS) 79-20006 (Washington, D.C., 1978).

4. The Social Security Act (Title II), 42 USC sec. 401. Social security benefit regulations are contained in Part 404 of Title 20 of the *Code of Federal Regulations*.

5. Commerce Clearing House, Inc, *1974 Social Security and Medicare Explained* (1974), and Charles I. Schottland, *The Social Security Program in the United States* (1970) (New York: Appleton, Century and Crofts).

6. U.S. Social Security Administration, *OASDI Digest*, DHEW Publication No. (SSA) 74-11917 (Washington, D.C.: Department of Health, Education and Welfare, 1974).

7. National Senior Citizens Law Center, *Materials on the Supplemental Security Income Program* (Los Angeles, December 1974).

8. Ibid.

9. James H. Schulz, *Pension Aspects of the Economics of Aging: Present and Future Roles of Private Pensions*. Committee Print, U.S. Senate Special Committee on Aging (Washington, D.C.: U.S. Government Printing Office, 1970). See also, Carter C. Osterbond, "Income in Retirement: The Need and Society's Responsibility" (A report on the 16th Annual Southern Conference on Gerontology) (Gainsville, Fla.: University of Florida Press, 1967); and Dorothy McCamman, "The Role of Private Pensions in Providing Retirement Income in the United States, *Income in Retirement*, 1975 (New York: Institute of Life Insurance), pp. 100-120.

10. *ERISA Simplification Act*, 1980, presented to U.S. 96th Cong., 2d session.

11. Roger F. Murray, "Economic Aspects of Pension: A Summary Report," *U.S. Joint Economic Committee, Old Age Income Assurance*, part V (Washington, D.C.: U.S. Government Printing Office, 1967).

12. Robert J. Myers, "Government and Pensions," *Private Pensions and the Public Interest* (Washington, D.C.: American Enterprise Institute for the Public Policy Research, 1970).

13. James H. Schulz, Guy Carrin, Hans Krupp, Manfred Peschke, Eliot Sclar, and J. Van Steenberge, *Providing Adequate Retirement Income-Pension Reform in the United States and Abroad* (Hanover, N.H.: Brandeis University Press/New England Press, 1974).

14. U.S. Department of Health, Education and Welfare, *Facts about Older Americans*.

15. James H. Schulz, *The Economics of Aging*, 2d ed. (Belmont, Calif.: Wadsworth Publishing Company, 1979.

16. U.S. Department of Agriculture, Food and Nutrition Service, *The Food Stamp Program* (Washington, D.C.), and U.S., Congress, Senate, Special Committee on Aging, *Hearing on Effectiveness of Food Stamps for Older Americans*, 19 April 1977 (Washington, D.C.: U.S. Government Printing Office, 1977).

17. Federal Council on the Aging, "The Impact of the Tax Structure on the Elderly" (Washington, D.C., December 1975).

18. Schulz, et al., *Providing Adequate Retirement*.

19. U.S., Congress, Senate, Special Committee on Aging, *Future Directions in Social Security—Unresolved Issues: An Interim Staff Report*, 1975.

20. U.S. Department of Health, Education and Welfare, Social Security Administration. *Social Security Programs Around the World* (Washington, D.C., 1973).

5 Health Policy and Programs

Health policy must take into account those problems that distinguish older people from the nonelderly. When applied to the elderly we are concerned not only with the elderly's access to treatment for specific illnesses but also with their need for a full array of health-related services that will help them remain in as good physical and mental health as possible and in the mainstream of community life. In addition, sufficient resources have to be secured for nutrition, health education, and biomedical research, because means for coping with chronic illness and disability have to be developed and dread diseases, which disproportionately affect older persons, have to be prevented.

Two Definitions of Health

In practice, health in the aged is usually defined in one of two ways: in terms of the presence or absence of disease or in terms of how well the older person is functioning. A definition of health in terms of pathology or disease is commonly used by health personnel, particularly physicians. This is a medical perspective on health. A judgment of health based on the presence or absence of pathology is the result of observation, examination, and the findings of laboratory tests.

An alternative way of defining health among the elderly is based not on pathology but on level of functioning. This perspective has been summarized by a World Health Organization Advisory group: " . . . health in the elderly is best measured in terms of function; . . . degree of fitness rather than extent of pathology may be used as a measure of the amount of services the aged will require from the community." The points of view of those who prefer the medical model of health needs and of those who prefer the functional model are not irreconcilable, and efforts have been made to assess the two models by comparing the self-reports of old people with the findings of physical examinations.[1]

Each person ages differently and the interaction between physical and mental health and between health and social and environmental factors all affect the measurement of "well-being" among the elderly. Rates of limitations in physical and emotional performance and on independent living, by age, are illustrated in table 5-1.

Table 5-1
Limitations of Performance and Independent Living by Age
(percent)

Category of Limitation	Age	Minimal Limitation	Some Limitation	Substantial Limitation	Severe Limitation
Physical	65-74	56.4	23.7	9.7	10.1
performance	75+	29.7	27.9	22.5	19.9
Emotional	65-74	32.1	35.2	22.6	10.1
performance	75+	25.5	39.3	22.2	12.9

	Age	None	Limited but Independent	Mobility Assistance Needed	Personal-Care Assistance Needed
Independent	65-74	77.4	11.1	8.5	3.0
living	75+	59.5	14.7	16.7	9.1

Source: U.S. Department of Health, Education and Welfare, Federal Council on Aging, *Public Policy and the Frail Elderly* (Washington, D.C., December 1978), p. 27.

The U.S. General Accounting Office (GAO) used the OARS multidimensional functional assessment survey instrument to determine the well-being status and impairment level of older persons in Cleveland as part of its study. GAO combined its data and material resulting from the development of the instrument at the OARS-Duke project (see table 5-2).[3] The OARS survey asks questions in five areas of human functioning: social, economic, mental, physical, and activities of daily living. The results in each area are combined to form a picture of overall well-being. The scale begins with "unimpaired," which means excellent or good in all five areas of human functioning. At the other end of the scale, "extremely impaired" means mild or moderate impairment in four areas and severe or complete impairment in the other, or complete impairment in two or more areas.[4]

As can be seen from table 5-3, the extremely impaired rate doubles between the 75 to 79 age group and the 80 to 84 age group. These data support a policy that there is a second older-age status, with the presumption of frailty at a certain advanced age, and therefore, a strategy of social intervention is needed to provide services for the frail elderly based on automatic entitlement.[5]

There are two major obstacles to promoting improvements in the elderly's health in the United States. One is the widely held belief that all the care needed can be supplied through the present system of medical care. The second obstacle is the escalating cost of medical care and any country's limited resources. Today's system of health care is mostly dictated by a medical ideology of short-term cure, applicable more to a younger population; an older population, particularly the frail elderly, increasingly

Table 5-2
Status of Well-Being by Institutionalization

Impairment Level	Noninstitutionalized People (%)	Institutionalized People (%)
Unimpaired	21	1
Slightly	21	1
Mildly	18	2
Moderately	17	5
Generally	9	4
Greatly	7	11
Extremely	7	76

Source: U.S. Department of Health, Education and Welfare, Federal Council on Aging, *Public Policy and the Frail Elderly* (Washington, D.C., December 1978), p. 28.

demands long-term care. Therefore, it does not make much sense to devote an increasing proportion of the country's health resources to medical treatment for illness on a short-term basis when the growth of the elderly population demands a greater concern with long-term care.

Health Status and Health Care Utilization

Chronic conditions are more prevalent among older persons than younger. In 1976, about 39 percent of older persons were limited in their major activity (working or keeping house) due to such conditions, as compared to only 7 percent for younger persons. In 1972, about 18 percent of the 65 + group had an interference with their mobility due to chronic conditions: 6 percent had some trouble getting around alone, 7 percent needed a

Table 5-3
Status of Well-Being by Age
percent

Well-Being Status	Under 70	70-74	75-79	80-84	85 +
Unimpaired	25.8	20.5	14.9	8.7	9.2
Slightly impaired	25.1	25.0	15.7	15.0	11.2
Mildly impaired	19.2	19.5	21.0	21.4	22.5
Moderately impaired	13.7	12.1	22.6	17.9	14.3
General impaired	5.4	10.8	9.3	11.6	12.2
Greatly impaired	1.9	2.9	3.6	2.9	2.0
Very greatly impaired	2.6	2.4	3.6	4.6	6.1
Extremely impaired	6.3	6.8	9.3	17.9	22.5

Source: U.S. Department of Health, Education and Welfare, Federal Council on Aging, *Public Policy and the Frail Elderly* (Washington, D.C., December 1978), p. 29.

mechanical aid to get around, and 5 percent were homebound. In 1976, older people had about a 1-in-6 chance of being hospitalized during a year, higher than for persons under 65 (1 in 10). Among those hospitalized during the year, the proportion with more than one stay was greater for older persons than for younger persons (26 percent versus 15 percent) and the average length of stay was about 5 days longer (11.6 versus 6.9 days). On the average, older people had more physician visits than did persons under 65 (6.9 versus 4.7 visits) in 1976, and a higher proportion had visited a doctor within the last 6 months (70 percent versus 58 percent).[6]

Growth of the Health Care Industry

In 1976, the nation spent $120 billion for personal health care. About $35 billion or 29 percent of this amount was spent for older persons, a rise from 8.2 billion in 1966 and an increase of 190 percent in real dollars. The per-capita health care cost for an older person was $1,738, nearly three times as much as the $547 spent for younger adults. Benefits from government programs, including medicare ($15.0 billion) and medicaid ($5.6 billion), accounted for about two-thirds of the health expenditures of older persons, as compared with three-tenths for adults under 65.[7]

Before medicare was enacted in 1966, 15 percent of health care expenditures was attributable to nursing-home costs; by 1977 that proportion had risen to 20 percent. Although medicare picked up 40 percent of the health care bill, the elderly were worse off because health costs had more than tripled by 1977.

Today's system of medical care, as shaped and directed by the medical profession, is concerned almost solely with the treatment of illness. Yet, health status is affected far more by such factors as education, nutrition, housing, personal hygiene, life-styles, environmental pollution, and working conditions than by medicine. Therefore, it makes no sense to devote an increasing proportion of the country's resources to medicine for the treatment of illness, especially when the amount of resources is increasingly limited.

Real growth in the nation's gross national product (GNP) during the current year may be only 2 to 3 percent. Yet, because of the economics of health care, diminished growth rates are not constraining the proportion of resources allocated to the treatment of illness. If more of these resources are to be allocated more to health-effective measures and less to purely medical care, the entire health industry will need to be restructured.

The present medical care system—the health industry—is one of the largest of the nation's economic sectors. Since medicare began, health spending has tripled, increasing at an annual rate of 12 percent. By 1977, this spending totalled $163 billion and accounted for 8.8 percent of GNP. Simultaneously, the proportion of this spending coming from public funds grew from 26 to 42 percent. Medicare and medicaid account for 60 percent of the entire federal health budget, and their costs are increasing at 15 percent a year.

If the rate of increase in spending for the treatment of illness is ever to be controlled (so that some resources can be "freed up" for use in ways having a greater impact on health status), one must understand why this economic sector has been growing so rapidly. This growth is due partly to the expansion of the elderly population. In 1976, although the elderly were only 11 percent of the population, they accounted for two-thirds of personal health care expenditures, 90 percent of hospital expenditures, and 60 percent of expenditures for physician services. This growing demand for medical services has been met partly through a 50 percent expansion of hospital capacity, hospital personnel, and health care professionals over the period 1960 to 1975.

Government has subsidized both the demand and supply sides of this growth. On the demand side, the private third-party payment system's growth has been subsidized through the tax laws. Also Blue Cross and Blue Shield are tax exempt in most states. Finally, the public medicare and medicaid programs were patterned after the private third-party payment system. On the supply side, hospital expansion was stimulated by the Hill-Burton program and by tax exemption of hospital-construction bonds. Federal spending for the training of health professionals totalled $5 billion between 1964 and 1976.

Government subsidies to increase the supply of medical facilities and services were expected to moderate costs for health care. However, the third-party payment system makes patients indifferent to cost, except the part for which they are responsible out-of-pocket. Consequently, there is little restraint on the rate of increase in charges of providers or the rate of increase in costs they incur. Third-party payers reimburse hospitals for virtually all costs incurred and cover much of the fees charged by physicians and other professionals. Also, doctors tend to overutilize hospitals, the most expensive component of the medical care system, and this overutilization is promoted by the third-party payment system, which tends to cover hospital services but not less costly out-of-hospital services.

As a consequence of this structure, medical costs and charges (and therefore total spending) have been growing much faster than prices in general. In the postwar period, price increases for the things medical care providers provide have accounted for about 55 percent of this growth, of which increases in technology account for about 35 percent and population increases account for about 10 percent.[8]

At this point it is useful to take a closer look at the two major governmental reimbursement mechanisms that have been designed to meet the financial costs of health care of older persons: medicare and medicaid.

Medicare

Medicare is a health-insurance program for the elderly sponsored by the federal government through the Social Security Administration, under Title XVIII of the Social Security Act. There are two parts to the medicare program: Part A, the hospital insurance component, which pays for hospital, skilled-nursing facility, and some home-health services; and Part B, the supplementary medical insurance component, which covers physician services, hospital outpatient services, and other forms of medical treatment. Part A benefits are automatically available without premium charges to those over 65 who qualify for social security or railroad retirement (and those under 65 who have received cash benefits based on disability for twenty-four months). Part B requires premium payments of $8.70 per month on the basis of the rate in effect through June 1980. The rate is subject to change each July 1.

Administration

Overall responsibility for the administration of medicare lies with the Health Care Financing Administration. The vast majority of medicare beneficiaries are also receiving social security old-age benefits. Part A of medicare, like social security, is funded by taxes on earnings of those currently employed or self-employed. (The small percentage of individuals who are age 65 or over and not eligible for social security or railroad retirement benefits may obtain Part-A coverage by paying a monthly premium.) Part B is paid in part by the monthly premiums of those insured and partly by federal contributions from general revenues.

The actual payment for medical services, however, is handled by private insurance organizations—such as Blue Cross—under contract to the federal government. Payments are made directly by the insurer (called the fiscal intermediary) to the hospital providing the care under Part A of medicare. Under Part B, the organization (called the "carrier" here) can make the payments directly to the individual beneficiary unless he has assigned his claim to the treating physician.

State agencies, under agreement with the SSA, have the responsibility of inspecting providers of medical services—hospitals, nursing homes, and home-health agencies—to ensure that they meet the conditions of participation in the Medicare program.

Eligibility

All persons over 65 who are entitled to social security or railroad retirement benefits or those who have received such benefits for more than twenty-four months based on their disability, are automatically eligible for medicare hospital insurance. Others may enroll within seven months of reaching age 65 by paying a monthly premium. There is also special coverage without premium charge for a limited group of individuals under age 65 who have severe kidney disease.

A beneficiary eligible for Part A of medicare is now automatically enrolled in Part B—the Supplementary Medical Insurance Program. The monthly premium is deducted from the monthly social security check unless the recipient elects to reject enrollment in the program. An individual who meets all requirements for social security benefits at age 65 but who cannot receive monthly payments because of continued earnings from employment or self-employment receives Part-A medicare coverage without payment of premiums by making application just the same as he would be were there no continued earnings.

Hospital Insurance—Part A of Medicare

The hospital-insurance component of medicare generally pays for hospital, nursing-home, and professional home-health care services. However, there are important deductions and limitations to the benefits.

Hospital Care. As of the present, medicare pays for up to ninety days of hospitalization per "spell of illness." A spell of illness has a special and precise definition under the law, usually called *benefit period*. It begins on the first day when hospital services are provided under Part A and ends when the person has gone sixty consecutive days without receiving inpatient hospital or skilled-nursing facility care covered under Part A. If the recipient suffers a relapse or requires rehospitalization for any other reason, a new benefit period begins, and the recipient is entitled to another ninety days of coverage.

Presently, the patient must pay for the first $144 of charges for hospitalization. Medicare assumes the rest of the cost for the first sixty days of the hospital stay. After the sixtieth day (and through the ninetieth day) the patient must contribute $36 a day as coinsurance. The amount of the deductible and coinsurance is subject to change each calendar year.

Every medicare recipient is also entitled to a lifetime reserve of sixty days of coverage. If the patient must remain in the hospital beyond the regular ninety-day period of medicare coverage during one benefit period, he or she may draw on this additional sixty days of lifetime reserve. This reserve period is nonrenewable. Once the sixty days are exhausted, there is no more additional reserve period. If the patient uses any of his lifetime reserve, he must contribute coinsurance, which during 1978 was $72 a day, one-half of the applicable daily rate.

For psychiatric hospital care, the beneficiary may receive 190 total days of care under Part A, but this is not renewable for each benefit period. So, after a beneficiary receives 190 days of psychiatric hospital care, he cannot receive any more Part A benefits for that type of care. Congress is now reviewing several of these provisions with an eye toward liberalization.

Nursing-Home Care. Medicare will pay for up to one hundred days of care in an approved skilled-nursing facility per benefit period. The patient must contribute $18 per day during the calendar year (in 1978) from the twenty-first to one-hundredth day. Patients must also meet four basic conditions to qualify for nursing-home payments: (1) they must have spent at least three days in a row in a hospital before their nursing-home stay; (2) they must have been admitted to the nursing facility within fourteen days of discharge from the hospital; (3) the reason for the stay in the nursing home was treated in a hospital; and (4) a doctor must certify that skilled-nursing treatment on a daily basis is medically necessary. Nursing-home care obtained because a person requires care for a serious ailment for which she or he has not just been hospitalized is not paid for by medicare.

Except for very limited emergency-hospital situations, the care must be obtained in a participating hospital and participating skilled-nursing facility. Most hospitals do participate, but many nursing homes do not. Medicare coverage includes all reasonable nursing-home expenses, including room and board, nursing care, physical therapy, and so on.

Home-Health Care. Hospital-insurance benefits may be paid for one hundred home-health visits by a visiting nurse or health worker during the twelve-month period following the patient's discharge from a hospital or nursing facility. The patient must have been hospitalized for at least three days and must have begun a home-health-care plan within fourteen days of discharge from a hospital or nursing home. The home-health-care plan must be periodically certified by a doctor, and its purpose must be to continue treatment for a condition that was previously treated in the hospital.

If the patient was not previously hospitalized, costs for one hundred home-health-care visits during a calendar year may be paid by the Part B medical-insurance plan. These visits must be obtained from a home-health agency that has been approved for participation in medicare.

Payments. Normally, the medicare patient, on admittance to the hospital or nursing facility and on billing, will sign a social security request-for-payment form. The institution then forwards billing forms directly to Blue Cross or another designated intermediary insurer.

The government—through the private-insurance intermediary—pays the hospital or skilled-nursing facility. The institution that provided the care must accept the medicare payment as payment in full for the institutional care (except for first day's deductible and the coinsurance). It cannot charge patients for any care covered by Part A beyond the patients' deductible and their coinsurance obligation, if any.

Supplementary Medical Insurance—Part B of Medicare

The supplementary-medical-insurance portion of medicare covers physician services, hospital-outpatient services, home-health care (in addition to that provided by Part A), diagnostic laboratory and X-ray services, and a variety of miscellaneous medical costs. The coverage is not total. In addition to the monthly premium, the medicare beneficiary must pay the first $60 of his or her annual medical expenses (for a calendar year) and generally at least 20 percent of the remaining expenses.

Covered Services. Covered services and material include the following:

1. Consultation, diagnosis, and surgery, whether performed in a doctor's office, hospital, or the patient's home, physician's services are covered. (There is a limit of 62.5 percent of cost for physician's psychiatric services rendered outside a hospital and not more than $250 of such cost for any calendar year will be reimbursed.)

2. Supplies and drugs furnished by a physician are covered. These must be part of the doctor's treatment. Drugs that can be self-administered are not covered.

3. Outpatient hospital services are covered—those services performed in a hospital on one who is not a full-time resident patient (for example, emergency room treatment).

4. Diagnostic laboratory tests, including X rays and other tests prescribed by a doctor, are covered.

5. Outpatient physical-therapy and speech-pathology services are covered.

6. Certain medical treatment supplies and equipment, including surgical dressings, casts, braces, prosthetic devices, and artificial limbs, are covered.

7. Rental or purchase of durable medical equipment, including wheelchairs, traction equipment, crutches, inhalators, and oxygen equipment, are covered.

8. Certain ambulance services are covered.

9. Home-health services are covered up to one-hundred visits a year if the patient is confined to his home and a doctor certifies that part-time

skilled-nursing care is necessary. The one-hundred-visit limitation is in addition to those covered by hospital insurance under Part A. Home-health-care services are paid for at 100 percent; there is no 20 percent coinsurance requirement as with the other services.

Payments. Generally, institutions providing Part-B medical services are reimbursed in the same manner as in Part-A coverage; that is, payments are made directly to the institution through the insurance carrier. There is a different procedure for private doctor bills. The individual beneficiary may be reimbursed directly, or he can assign the right to claim benefits to his physician (who then bills the insurance carrier).

Payments for physician's services are based on "reasonable charges," which are the lower of: (1) the customary fee charged by the physician; or (2) the seventy-fifth percentile of the prevailing charge for similar services in the physician's area.

If the physician accepts assignment, he must accept the medicare payment together with the patient's 20 percent contribution as full payment for his services. If the physician does not accept assignment or if the patient chooses not to make the assignment, medicare pays the patient 80 percent of the reasonable charges for the services, and the patient is liable for the doctor's bill even if it is considerably higher than the reasonable charges on which the medicare payment is based.

Recent figures have shown that about 50 percent of physicians treating medicare patients accept assignment of medicare claims. Although doctors might receive a smaller fee by receiving payment from the medicare insurer, the payment is quicker and surer than by billing the patient. This is especially true because when the medicare payment is made to the patient—that is, when there is no assignment—the patient does not have to show that he has paid the doctor. Thus, he may obtain the payment on the basis of an unpaid physician's bill.

Services Excluded from Medicare Coverage

Services not covered by medicare insurance include: services and supplies that are "not reasonable and necessary for the diagnosis and treatment of illness or injury"; custodial care, that is, care requiring less than daily skilled-nursing services; services paid for by a government agency (other than under medicare), such as care in a Veterans Administration facility or care paid for by the military Civilian Health and Medical Program (CHAMPUS); routine physical examinations; prescription and nonprescription drugs and medicines (except those administered in a hospital or by a physician); eyeglasses and examinations to fit glasses; hearing aids and examinations for hearing aids; dentures and routine dental treatment; orthopedic shoes, supportive devices for the feet, and treatment for flat feet; immunizations; cosmetic surgery.

Most of the noncovered services are specific and easily identifiable. Certain exclusions however, are more vague and have given rise to much court litigation. The custodial-care definition has been especially troublesome, and the SSA has been reversed by courts numerous times for using it to deny medicare payments to patients in nursing homes.[9] Table 5-4 presents a schematic overview of medicare benefits as of 1980.

Medicaid

Medicaid, established in 1965 under the Social Security Act Title XIX, is a cooperative federal-state medical-assistance program for the needy poor. Unlike medicare, medicaid is a welfare program rather than an insurance program. And unlike medicare, eligibility for medicaid is based on proven need. Medicaid, like medicare, pays for a broad range of medical services, and actually the scope of covered services is considerably broader than under medicare.

Medicaid is funded jointly by the federal government and state governments, the amount of the federal contribution to states varying from 50 percent fo 83 percent. There are federal guidelines for the program, but the responsibility for its administration lies with state agencies. The application process and most of the individual, day-to-day administration is handled by local and county welfare offices. As with medicare, payment of medicaid claims in many states is handled by private insurance organizations.

Eligibility

Eligibility criteria for medicaid and the range of available services vary from state to state, but there are some general principles that apply to all states. As a rule, aged (over 65), blind, and disabled persons receiving supplementary-security income (SSI) and their essential spouses are eligible for medicaid. (An *essential spouse* is the husband or wife of an aged, blind, or disabled public-assistance recipient. The spouse must be living with the recipient and his or her care must be necessary to the well-being of the recipient. Also, the spouse must have been treated as "essential" by the state law prior to January 1974.) However, states can adopt welfare criteria employed before SSI took effect, so it is possible in a few states for a person to be eligible for SSI but not for medicaid. Families receiving Aid for Families with Dependent Children (AFDC) automatically qualify for medicaid.

Table 5-4
Medicare Chart

Service	Benefit	Medicare Pays	You Pay
		For Covered Services—Each Benefit Period	
Part A (Hospital Insurance)			
Hospitalization: Semiprivate room and board, general nursing and miscellaneous hospital services and supplies.	First 60 days	All but $180	$180
	61st to 90th day	All but $45 a day	$45 a day
	91st to 150th day[b]	All but $90 a day	$90 a day
Includes meals, special care units, drugs, lab tests, diagnostic X-rays, medical supplies, operating and recovery room, anesthesia and rehabilitation services.	Beyond 150 days	Nothing	All costs
A Benefit Period begins on the first day you receive services as an inpatient in a hospital and ends after you have been out of the hospital or skilled nursing facility for 60 days in a row.			
Posthospital skilled-nursing-facility care: In a facility approved by Medicare. You must have been in a hospital for at least 3 days and enter the facility within 14 days after hospital discharge.	First 20 days	100% of reasonable costs	Nothing
	Additional 80 days	All but $22.50/Day	$22.50/Day
	Beyond 100 days	Nothing	All costs
Medicare and private insurance will not pay for most nursing home care. You pay for custodial care and most care in a nursing home.			
Posthospital home-health care	Up to 100 visits	100% of reasonable costs	Nothing
Blood	Blood	All but first 3 pints	For first 3 pints

Part B (Medical Insurance)

Service		Medicare Pays	You Pay
Medical expense: Physician's services, inpatient and outpatient medical services and supplies, physical and speech therapy, ambulance, etc.	Medicare pays for medical services in or out of hospital. Some insurance policies pay less (or nothing) for hospital out-patient medical services or services in a doctor's office	80% of reasonable charge (after $60 deductible)	$60 deductible[c] plus 20% of balance of reasonable charge (plus any charge above reasonable)[d]
Home-health care	Up to 100 visits	100% of reasonable charge (after $60 deductible)	Subject to deductible[c]
Outpatient hospital treatment	Unlimited as medically necessary	80% of reasonable charge (after $60 deductible)	Subject to deductible[c] plus 20% of balance of reasonable charge[d]
Blood	Blood	80% of reasonable charge (after first 3 pints)	For first 3 pints plus 20% of balance of reasonable charge[d]

[a] These figures are for 1979 and are subject to change each year.

[b] 60 Lifetime Reserve Days may be used only once; days used are not renewable.

[c] Once you have had $60 of expense for covered services in a calendar year, the Part-B deductible does not apply to any further covered services you receive in that year.

[d] You pay for charges higher than reasonable charges allowed by Medicare unless the doctor or supplier agrees to accept Medicare's reasonable charge as the total charge for services rendered.

Categorically Needy. Medicaid coverage of the categorically needy—those receiving SSI or some form of public assistance—is required by federal law, if the state elects to have a medicaid program. As has been noted, the income levels of those considered categorically needy vary according to the state.

Medically Needy. States, at their option, may also provide medicaid coverage to another group—the medically needy. The medically needy are persons who have income and resources in excess of the limits necessary to qualify for welfare but who are still unable to pay their medical expenses. To qualify, a person must have incurred medical obligations that reduce his income below the welfare standard. About half of the states now provide medicaid coverage to this medically needy group.

Application

Application for medicaid is part of the state welfare-application process. One usually applies at a local or county welfare office. The state agency is obligated to furnish all medicaid applicants with full information about the program and the particular benefits available to them. Medicaid cards are issued as evidence of eligibility. In some states, new cards are issued every month, containing labels limiting the number of services available in a one-month period.

Applications are supposed to be processed promptly, within forty-five days, or sixty days if disability is involved. Eligibility dates from the first of the month of application. States must pay for all covered medical services rendered to the applicant during the three months prior to the application (assuming that the applicant could have been eligible during those three months).

Benefits

Range of Services. Benefits available under medicaid vary greatly from state to state. There are, however, certain basic mandatory services for which every state must pay, at least for persons receiving AFDC or SSI. These essential services include: (1) inpatient hospital services; (2) outpatient hospital services; (3) physician services, whether rendered in an office, hospital, nursing facility, or patient's home; (4) X rays and laboratory services; (5) skilled-nursing-home services. Medicaid must also pay for a recipient's transportation if it is necessary to secure medical care.

In addition to these five required services, there is a list of further services that states, at their option, may offer. These optional benefits include: home-health care and private-nursing services; dental care and treatment and dentures; physical therapy and related services; prescription drugs; eyeglasses and hearing aids; mental hospital care to those over 65; prosthetic devices. Currently, several states under budgetary constraints and "Proposition 13 fever" are proposing to eliminate or cut back on many of these benefits.

In many states, prior authorization from the state agency administering the medicaid program is required before a recipient can accept the available services. For example, authorization is often required before a medicaid patient can undergo surgery, receive nonroutine dental care, or rent medical equipment.

The medicaid recipient has full freedom of choice to select the institution or physician as provider of medical services. Physicians, however, are not required to accept medicaid patients. In fact, many physicians prefer not to take medicaid cases because of the relatively low fee schedules, complex billing procedures, and other bureaucratic requirements. In some areas, nonavailability of physicians is a major problem for medicare and medicaid recipients.

Amount and Duration of Services. States have wide discretion to limit the amount and duration of medical services as well as the scope of offered services. The only requirements under federal law are that each state specify in advance the amount and/or duration of each particular service available to the medicaid recipient and that the amount and/or duration be sufficient to "reasonably achieve" the purpose of the service. What this means is that states can and do limit hospital stays, for example, to thirty days per year or physician visits to two a month. State limitations that are unduly restrictive have been challenged in court as not meeting the federal standard of reasonable medical care (for example, Louisiana formerly limited medicaid payments to one physician visit a month for patients with chronic illness, and Georgia limited hospital stays to ten days per stay).

Payment

Billing. Bills for medicaid services are submitted by the provider of the services to the state agency (or insurance carrier) for payment. Hospitals are reimbursed on a reasonable-cost basis, often in the same manner as under medicare. Payment for physician's services is on a reasonable-charge basis, but the system used to arrive at this figure varies widely from state to state. Some states use the medicare standard of the seventy-fifth percentile of prevailing charges in the area; others follow private-insurance fee policies with generally higher compensation rates; still others impose their own fee schedules, often at considerably lower rates than the physician would normally charge.

Both physicians and institutions must accept the medicaid payment as full reimbursement for their services. They cannot bill the medicaid patient in addition (except to collect the modest copayments required for certain services in some states).

Deductibles. The copayments or deductibles required in some states cannot be imposed on AFDC or SSI recipients for the five mandatory medicaid services, which include hospital, skilled-nursing facility, and physician services. Deductibles can, however, be required of the medically needy for all services. And deductibles can be required of all beneficiaries for nonmandatory services. The deductibles are usually small token contributions—for example, a $1 payment for each time a prescription is filled.

Premiums. In addition, all states impose an income-related premium on the medically needy. The premium is a fixed sum—usually $1 or $2 dollars—which the Medicaid recipient must pay on a monthly or quarterly basis whether or not he or she uses medicaid services.

Hearings and Appeals

All states are required to provide fair hearing and appeal procedures to medicaid applicants and recipients. Persons who have been denied initial enrollment in the medicaid program, those who are denied further benefits, and those who have been denied coverage for a particular service all have a right to challenge the administrative decisions at a hearing.

The hearings, like those conducted by the Social Security Administration (SSA) in OASDI and SSI cases, should have most protections required for fair hearings, for the individual petitioner has the right to personally appear at the hearing, to be represented by an attorney, and to submit oral and written evidence.

Beyond the hearing stage, there should be some right to a further administrative appeal, usually to the state agency in charge of the medicaid program. Of course, judicial review, either in federal or state court (depending on the issue raised) is available once the administrative appeal course is completed.[10]

Long-Term Care

Long-term care consists of those services designed to offer diagnostic, preventive, therapeutic, rehabilitative, supportive, and maintenance services for individuals of all age groups who have chronic physical, developmental, or emotional impairments. This care is provided in a variety of institutional and noninstitutional health and social care settings, including the home, with the goal of promoting the optimum level of physical, social, and psychological functioning.

Medical advances, especially in the areas of emergency medicine, pediatrics, psychiatry, and geriatrics have underscored the importance of long-term-care services stemming from the fact that persons of all ages now survive illnesses and trauma that would have once been fatal. Survival is often accompanied by extremely limited capabilities for independent functioning and living, which results in the need for coordinated care among a variety of institutions and programs, both private and public.

The lack of long-term-care systems that encompass both health and social services is the greatest deficiency in the present health structure from an elderly viewpoint. The elderly's access to long-term care is restricted by the nonavailability of services and qualified personnel and by their financial inability to pay for those services even if they are available.

The implications of demographic trends for long-term-care policy is significant, since the elderly have the highest incidence of functional disability. Demand for long-term-care service is going to increase rapidly. Yet, current demand is not even being met. Of 8 million persons estimated to be in need of assistance with daily activities in 1975, only 2.3 million received long-term care under government programs. Over half of nursing-home costs in 1975 were paid from private sources; 44 percent of these costs were paid for out-of-pocket. The average annual cost of nursing-home stay in that year was $7,300. It is no wonder that nursing home care is the main "catastrophic" health expense of the elderly. They are forced to deplete their resources or "spend down" (impoverish themselves) to become eligible for medicaid assistance for nursing homes.

The financial difficulties of medicare and medicaid inhibit significant expansion of long-term-care services. Meanwhile, the costs are being driven up by high inflation, demographic trends, and increased utilization of services. The combined effect has been a doubling of total (government and private) spending for long-term care from approximately $11 billion in 1975 to an estimated $28 billion in 1980.[11]

Conditions and Problems of Long-Term Care

Too many of those who have required long-term care have been cared for in large isolated institutions apart from the rest of society. They have often been placed in facilities for the mentally ill or developmentally disabled, frequently understaffed and often lacking adequately trained personnel. Deinstitutionalization per se is not the solution. Shortcomings in institution-based care are paralleled by the absence of a viable system of community long-term care. Needed is a continuum of care and services, with a range of options based on the needs of those who require care. Financial barriers and eligibility regulations are adding to fragmentation and discrimination in the access to services. Frequently our major shortcoming is that the family—which provides the primary support system—lacks the necessary buttressing options and supports that would strengthen its capacity to meet the social, emotional, and physical demands placed on it by the member in need of long-term care. Problems are often further complicated by the lack of knowledge on the part of the public about gaining access to adequate care and the ability to assess what is good care.

Long-term care for the aged in the United States is overly dependent on the nursing home. This hospitallike model for long-term care is particularly inappropriate, since it imposes a medical solution on a variety of social problems. An adequate long-term-care program requires a range of resources in the community as well as in institutions; sheltered-housing options seem a desirable alternative to the nursing home.

Presently five major problems occur in long-term-care programs, even in countries that have better developed systems than the United States.

1. Accelerating costs within a finite set of national health and social service resources produce budgetary strain, particularly in inflationary times. With universal entitlements, the only means to control costs are to limit access, to recruit voluntary labor, or both. Bottlenecks develop that impede an easy flow of patients between acute hospital, old-age home, chronic hospital, and sheltered housing.

2. With the recognition of long-term care as a social rather than a medical problem, social service departments are responsible for some institutional care, day-care centers, and the home help and personal social services underpinning home health. Communication and coordination between health and social service departments on a local level is often a problem, notably in England.

3. The style of care varies greatly with the auspices of care. When care is viewed in the medical domain, emphasis is placed on more traditional diagnostic and treatment activities with relatively little attention paid to the problems of personal comfort and adaptation. On the other hand, the social service-operated institutions tend to pay far more attention to the personal comfort of patients and tend to be more reconciled to more supportive and less rehabilitative goals for patients.

4. Although greater equalization of financial rewards has reduced some of the turnover of personnel characterizing nursing homes, selection and training of staff is a continuous problem. In rural areas, with prevailing wage rates, it is even more difficult to retain the staff necessary to mount adequate home-health and day-care programs, nor do these areas generate the revenue necessary to support the full range of desired service unless heavily subsidized by the national treasury.

5. Reliable and valid data available to identify those programs that are effective in terms of reducing mortality and morbidity or improving the quality of patient life, or both, are few and far between. Without basic information about treatment and care effectiveness, it is impossible to discuss the relative cost-effectiveness of various noninstitutional programs such as home care and community-based programs as compared to institutional programs.[12]

As nursing homes constitute a sizeable segment of long-term-care programs for the elderly, let us take a look at the nature, cost, and funding of this type of institution.

Nursing Homes

Although the dictionary defines the term *nursing home* as "a hospital for convalescent or aged people," nursing homes, in actuality, bear little resemblance to hospitals in terms of medical, surgical, psychiatric, or rehabilitative services. A nursing home is primarily a residential facility with a minimal level of nursing care, designed for the convalescence and long-term care of the seriously ill of all ages, but primarily the aged. The public tends to include all residential-care facilities for the old under the term nursing home, but distinctions must be made on the basis of several factors, including ownershp (profit versus nonprofit), participation in federal reimbursement programs (medicare and medicaid), levels of care provided, and regulation by state licensing authorities.

The most common classification of nursing homes is based on the level of care they are able to provide. The skilled-nursing facility (SNF) provides the highest level of care, skilled nursing on a twenty-four-hour-a-day basis. The intermediate-care facility (ICF) provides supportive care and nursing services but not to the extent that an SNF does. This classification scheme is important to bear in mind when dealing with nursing homes that participate in federal reimbursement programs

A third type of long-term-care facility that is not a nursing home at all is the residential care home. Also known as board-and-care homes or personal-care homes, these facilities do not provide medical or nursing care, are not eligible to participate in the medicare or medicaid programs, and are often unregulated by the states in which they operate. They normally provide group living arrangements and some assistance with daily needs such as bathing, food preparation, and eating.

Numbers and Auspice. As of now there are 25 percent more nursing-home beds in the United States than general and surgical hospital beds. There are more than three times as many nursing homes than hospitals; almost 50 percent more in-patient days of care are given each year in long-term care facilities than in short-term general hospitals; since 1972, medicaid expenditures for nursing-home care exceeded payments to general and surgical hospitals.

There are approximately 24 thousand nursing homes nationwide. Eight percent are operated by governmental entities (cities, counties, and states), 17 percent by nonprofit organizations such as religious groups and fraternal orders, and 75 percent are operated for profit. These figures, by themselves, indicate nothing about the quality of care provided. About 80 percent of the older persons in nursing homes reside in for-profit or commercial homes. Commercial nursing homes illustrate the potential conflict between profit and service in the care of the aged. Because of the predominance of commercial homes and their profit nature, most problems regarding quality of care occur with this group.

It is often difficult to determine who is actually responsible for the operation of a commercial nursing home. The owner may or may not be qualified to act as administrator under state law but can and usually does control the finances of the nursing home. The owners might be individuals, partnerships, or corporations with little or no interest in the day-to-day operation of the facility, who reserve themselves the authority to expend money for staff training, rehabilitative equipment, or food. Federal law requires nursing-home administrators to be licensed. There is no licensing requirement for owners. However, federal regulations require disclosure of ownership interests of 10 percent or more as well as the names of officers, directors or partners. (This information should be available at the offices of state departments of health.)

State Requirements. Nursing homes are required to be licensed by the state. The standards for licensure vary from state to state. In many states, residential-care facilities are not covered by the licensing requirement, although for the protection of older persons they should be. Recently there has been a trend to regulate such facilities. States may also license nursing-home personnel, including administrators, nurses, physical therapists, dieticians, and so on. In addition, local governments may have ordinances with which nursing homes are required to comply.

Inspections and licensing functions may be delegated to various agencies within a state. Though the breakdown varies from state to state, the fragmentation might consist of different agencies with authority to inspect and license, reimburse the facility, assign residents, and institute the procedures to close the facility. It is very important to learn who does what within each state, for where such fragmentation occurs, no single body can be responsible for the deficiencies in nursing-home-regulation enforcement. It is also essential to learn what enforcement mechanisms exist in each state to ensure compliance with state laws. These mechanisms may include loss of license, fines, or criminal penalties.

Federal Requirements. Federal regulations are applicable only where there is federal financial participation in payment of nursing-home costs. Thus, only those nursing homes that participate in medicare or medicaid must comply with federal standards.

Medicare covers only skilled-nursing facilities and pays a total of 7 percent of the nation's nursing-home bills; approximately forty-five hundred of the nation's twenty-four thousand nursing homes are medicare participants. To receive medicare reimbursements, the facility must be certified by complying with federal-regulation standards. These facilities must also be in compliance with the Life Safety Code of the National Fire Protection Association, as well as state and local regulations. The state standards are usually not as high, so that a home meeting the federal standards will almost always be in compliance with the state requirements.

As stated before, medicare operates uniformly across the nation by the federal government, and medicaid is a joint federal-state program whose benefits to the financially needy vary from state to state. Administered by the state under broad federal guidelines, medicaid encompasses two categories of persons—those that are categorically needy or receiving AFDC and SSI and those that are medically needy or persons whose assets and income exceed AFDC- or SSI-eligibility standards but lack sufficient resources to pay for the necessary medical care. Medicaid pays over 60 percent of the nursing-home bills, with seven thousand of the twenty-four thousand nursing homes as participants.

Since 1972 the requirements for both medicare and medicaid certification have been the same. In addition to meeting the federal standards, medicaid participants must also comply with the Life Safety Code and state and local requirements.

Federal Payments under Medicare and Medicaid. Medicare will pay for up to one hundred days of care in a "single spell of illness," which begins with hospital admission and ends sixty days after the last medicare-covered treatment. The person must have been hospitalized for at least three days and transferred to a nursing home within fourteen days after being released from the hospital. If space is not available in a nursing home within fourteen days, the time will be extended to twenty-eight days.

Not only does medicaid eligibility vary from state to state, but also the amount of coverage for nursing-home care varies. If a person qualifies for both medicaid and medicare, medicaid will pay the medicare premium, deductible, and coinsurance payments. The states are required by federal regulations to provide SNF care to medicaid-eligible recipients, but they may additionally choose to provide ICF care and to extend the coverage to medically needy medicaid recipients. Furthermore, as opposed to medicare, most states place no duration limits on medicaid-reimbursed care.

To be eligible for medicare or medicaid benefits, the recipient must be in need of the "level of care" covered by the program. To determine that the patient is receiving the proper level of care, the programs require (1) a physician certification stating that the care is medically necessary, and (2) a utilization review committee functioning within the nursing home to periodically review the patient's continuing need for the level of care provided by the facility. This mechanism serves as a means of cost control, assuring that neither medicare nor medicaid is paying for unnecessary care. Program review teams and professional standard review organizations (PSROs) also have been implemented to assure that the facility is supplying the required level of care. But this also results in a transferring of patients when it is determined that he or she no longer needs the level of care provided.

Standard Enforcement. In 1974, Senator Moss's Subcommittee on Long-Term Care determined that "it is conceivable that every nursing home in the nation violates at least one of the many applicable standards" and furthermore that over 50 percent of the nursing homes in the United States are substandard to the extent that "they have serious and life threatening (as opposed to technical) violations." Much of this can be attributed to an inefficient enforcement mechanism which can cause even the highest standards to be ineffective. The enforcement of regulations is left to the states.

There is no direct federal enforcement even of federal standards, which only apply to medicare or medicaid participants. The federal government's only sanction on noncomplying homes is to decertify them, thus stopping their medicare and medicaid reimbursements. When a nursing home is in compliance with federal regulations for certification, it is said to have a valid "provider agreement," which lasts for one year. This procedure guarantees an annual review, but even this does not assure that the home is constantly in compliance, for there are waivers and extensions in the law that allow a noncomplying home to continue its operations. When a nursing home is not in full compliance with federal regulations, it must prepare a "plan of correction," which is sent to the appropriate agency together with the inspection report to determine certification eligibility.

Recently, this all-or-nothing approach is being supplemented by a citation sytem whereby the nursing home is fined so much per violation per day depending on the severity of the violation. As of this writing, California, Florida, and Wisconsin are a few of the states that have instituted this system, which allows the nursing home to remain functioning, yet makes it financially unprofitable not to correct violations. Many of the statutes mandate that the nursing home post the citations received, an added incentive to meet the standards.

Advance notice of inspections and fragmentation of nursing-home responsibilities among various agencies within a state add to the inefficiency of any enforcement procedure. Recent legislation, such as that in California, Michigan, and Rhode Island, has prohibited advance notice of inspections so that a home will not as readily be able to effect a temporary cover up of its deficiencies.

Public Access to Information. If the nursing home is not a medicare/medicaid participant, the ability to review inspection reports depends on state law. Some states have disclosure provisions similar to the Freedom of Information Act, which will require that such reports be made available on request. To find out if such a law exists within a particular state, inquire at the office in charge of nursing-home licensure.

For nursing homes that participate in the medicare or medicaid programs, a 1972 amendment to the Social Security Act requires that inspection reports be made available to the public.

Rights of Nursing-Home Patients. A person does not give up any of his or her civil rights when he or she enters a nursing home. Even so, because of his or her physical and/or mental condition, the resident may be in a very vulnerable position. Some homes require that patients sign a life-care contract, whereby the patients turn over all their assets for a promise that they will be cared for until their death. Not only does this deprive the patient of any further bargaining power, but his or her longevity is not in the economic interest of the home. Because of this, some states have made the life-care contract illegal, and others have regulated its use. To the patient's advantage, some states require that a service contract be signed. This delineates the services provided and the costs charged, so that both the nursing home and patient know what is to be expected.

To further insure that the nursing-home patient retains his or her rights, the federal government has recently promulgated a patient's bill of rights, which applies to all medicare and medicaid homes. Skilled-nursing facilities and intermediate-care facilities each have their own patient's bill of rights, which vary only slightly.

The regulations require that the patients be informed of their rights and that the facility must establish a procedure and train their staff to implement them. Some of the provisions in the bill of rights call for the right to know and make decisions about one's treatment, the right to privacy and to confer with persons of his or her choice, and the right to voice grievances without fear of reprisal. The bill also prohibits transfers except for medical reasons, the patient's own welfare, or that of other patients, or for nonpayment. The bill further requires that nursing homes disclose all charges and fees and gives patients the right to manage their own finances and stipulates that they be given a quarterly accounting of the financial transactions made on their behalf by the nursing home if they have delegated that responsibility in writing.

There is no automatic-enforcement mechanism built into the patients' bill of rights, which might cut down on its effectiveness. As of now, the patient is left to assert his or her own rights, which could result in costly, time-consuming litigation.

Since the federal nursing-home patients' bill of rights covers only medicare and/or medicaid participants, there is the need for states to enact similar legislation so that all patients are covered. More and more states are doing this.

Nursing-Home *Ombudsmen. Ombudsman* is a Scandinavian term. Originally, the *ombudsman* was a government official, as in Sweden, who received complaints and suggestions and attempted to resolve them.

Between 1972 and 1975, HEW funded seven nursing-home ombudsman demonstration projects. They were to establish effective and viable mechanisms for receipt and resolution of complaints, as well as to document the long-term-care system and to bring about improvement within it. In 1975, HEW, through the Administration on Aging, funded smaller projects in each of the fifty states. Through this program, each state is to hire a "nursing home developmental specialist" who is to develop a process whereby the complaint receipt and resolution is to be done by volunteers at the "grass root" level (see chapter 7).[13]

Deinstitutionalization was the big push in the 1970s. Searches for alternatives to institutional care have elicited innumerable proposals to provide community-based care and to avoid "warehousing" the elderly. But it has not worked much better here than when deinstitutionalization was instituted for the mentally ill. Arthur J. Naparstek, professor of public administration at the University of Southern California, and David E. Biegel, director of that university's neighborhood and family-services project, came to the following conclusion:

> Federal mental health planners envisioned the flowering of a network of support services to care for deinstitutionalized patients at the community level through the stimulus of Federal seed money. But 1,300 of the 2,000 community mental health centers projected for 1980 have failed to materialize and many that did have failed to service this chronically ill population. Deinstitutionalization, an ostensibly humane treatment program, has degenerated into a tragic crisis. Public scrutiny of the situation needs to begin now. Planners, without real consultation, assumed that strong communities would accept the chronically ill. When few welcomed large numbers of these troubled people, patients were steered to transitional neighborhoods that would not put up a fuss, but the strong

community-support factor essential for successful aftercare was absent. The result was that city streets became wards of mental hospitals, and it was out of the snakepits and into the gutter for victims of the deinstitutionalization policy.[14]

Although home-care and day-care programs for the aged have been buffers against the excesses of a wholesale deinstitutionalization policy, they have, by no means, been given the financial, political, and social supports to become viable alternatives, and a policy to avoid unnecessary and uncalled-for warehousing of older persons has not yet been formulated that can be translated into action.[15]

Nutrition

The President's 1970 Task Force on Aging studied the nutritional needs of the elderly as a major ingredient of good health. In examining the incidence of malnutrition among the elderly, the Task Force concluded that insufficient income was only one of several causes. The lonely older person who can afford an adequate diet but does not eat properly; the older person who finds going to the store too great a burden; the older person who is nutritionally ignorant; the chronically ill older person unable to prepare a hot meal—all are part of the problem. The Task Force believes that programs can be designed that not only provide adequate nutrition to older persons, but equally important, combat their loneliness, channel them into the community, educate them about proper nutrition, and afford some of them an opportunity for paid community services. The Task Force recommended that the president direct the Administration on Aging and the Department of Agriculture to develop a program of technical assistance and financial assistance to local groups so they can provide daily meals and group dining to the many aged who need them and "meals on wheels" to the homebound. Such programs would not only meet nutritional needs, they would also provide meaningful employment and voluntary service for the healthy aged who are looking for work and are discriminated against in the job market. Moreover, older people gain immeasurably from the social setting of communal dining.[16]

The Administration on Aging conducted thirty-two research demonstrations in nutrition projects for the aged between 1968 and 1971. These pilot programs were considered very successful and helped advance the passage of congressional legislation for a nutrition program for the elderly. One hundred million dollars was to be available for the fiscal year 1973 and $150 million for fiscal year 1974. An estimated 250,000 older people would benefit, but there are more than 5 million persons over 60 years of age who would actually qualify for the program.

Most food programs had been legislated by the House and Senate agriculture committees and administered under the Department of Agriculture. The House and Senate agriculture committees have consistently dragged their feet on all nutritional and food proposals until Title VII of the Older American Act was passed in 1973 and finally incorporated into Title III in 1978.[17]

A Pilot Project to Demonstrate Alternative Health Services

The Alternative Health Services (AHS) program is a demonstration effort started in 1976 to serve clients in a seventeen-county area who are medicaid eligible, at least 50 years of age, and meet the state medicaid eligibility requirements for nursing-home care. It was initiated to provide services to the elderly so that they could remain in their own homes or return to community living from a nursing home. Home-delivered services (social support, homemaker, transportation, and so on), sheltered housing, and adult day rehabilitation are available to each client.

Projects in Georgia, Virginia, and New York are part of a national effort to counteract the current bias in public support for institutionally based long-term care. Ninety percent of all public funds for long-term care now go to nursing homes and 3 percent support residents in other institutions; only 7 percent finance community-based care. Most of this public institutional support comes from medicaid, which in 1978 financed 46 percent of the total national nursing-home bill of $15.751 billion. During this same year, medicaid paid only $211 million or roughly 1 percent of its budget of $18.613 billion for home-health care.

Historically, the bulk of public spending for long-term care has been funneled through medical programs for institutionally based services, even though the predominant need of the chronically impaired elderly has always been for social, residential, and health and medical services in the community. The passage of medicare and medicaid in 1965 continued this trend; the medical model in long-term care has been and still is dominant.

In 1979, the General Accounting Office (GAO) issued a report to Congress that outlines those problems in the current long-term-care system due to its focus on a medical model and its heavy bias toward institutional care. It also describes projects like the one in Georgia, and states the need for a stable funding source if AHS and similar programs are to become permanent components of the health and social service delivery system.

The report includes several major recommendations to Congress designed to increase the choices of older people when they need long-term care and to provide more public support for noninstitutional long-term care.

One of the recommendations proposes establishing a preadmission screening program that would encompass a comprehensive health and social assessment and a case-management component to monitor the services provided.

The report became the basis for a congressional hearing on "Community Based Care: Obstacles and Opportunities." The Select Committe on Aging subsequently introduced the Medicaid Community Care Act of 1980. This bill, which incorporates in part the recommendations in the GAO report, would increase the federal matching funds under medicaid by 25 percent for community-based services if the state agreed to provide a comprehensive medical and social assessment for nursing-home applicants. It also provides for an expanded range of home and community services and would increase the number of elderly who could be covered.

There is also a lot of interest in long-term-care reform in the Senate. The Senate Finance Committee staff have been at work on a legislative proposal that they are calling Title XXI. This new title to the Social Security Act would consolidate home-health services currently covered under medicare, medicaid, and Title XX under a new community-based long-term-care system that would serve all elderly.

What has been key to both House and Senate efforts is that there is recognition that shifts are needed in long-term care away from the current medical focus to a health and social system that is community oriented. Such a system would most likely mean that the role of the social work profession will be expanded as new services are developed and systems to coordinate these services are instituted and managed.[18]

Mental Health

Mental health needs to be viewed from two perpsectives: a treatment perspective that focuses on restoration and rehabilitation of older people who have mental impairments or who are classified and categorized as emotionally disturbed or mentally ill—this focus follows the medical model. A public health perspective, which concentrates on prevention, focuses on the environment and attempts to shape it to achieve mental health.

At the beginning of the twentieth century, one of the views held by psychiatrists on the nature of mental illness was that it was a symptom of inherent organic condition, offering little hope for recovery. The supporters of this view saw their role as providing isolated and custodial care to keep these people from public view. Almost eighty years later, remnants of this philosophy are still present.

In the early 1900s, state and county mental hospitals were built up and housed 150,151 persons, with the largest number of residents in 1955—

633,504. During this time, the older a person, the higher the rate of admission to a mental hospital. The care was custodial, offering little or no treatment. After World War II, the practice of mental health emphasized a treatment approach and acknowledged that much of the traditional backward chronicity was due to the hospitalization itself, which taught the patient to learn and act the sick role.

New approaches to patient care were implemented that attempted to minimize the alienation of patients from their social contacts and to introduce various alternatives to institutions such as day hospitals and community mental health centers, with varying degrees of success. However, most of the aged mentally ill are not receiving even the limited benefits of the more recent developments in mental health care. Although only 5 percent of the elderly are in institutions, over 30 percent of the mental hospital population is over 65, despite the fact that they are being moved in increasing numbers to nursing homes. This 30 percent figure is not made up primarily of those who have grown old in the hospital, but first admission rates for the 65 and over population are more than double that for the entire population. Less than 5 percent of the elderly make use of community mental health centers (CMHCs), and less than 2 percent are treated privately.

Kahn points out that the new mental health ideology had disproportional effects on different age groups. Before World War II, with custodialism as prevalent philosophy, older persons were more frequently hospitalized than the younger population. When the emphasis was placed on the therapeutic approach, only the young benefited from such treatment. For the aged, custodialism still existed; but they were shifted to nursing homes where no psychiatric services were available. In 1963, 53 percent of the aged mentally ill were in nursing homes and in 1969 the figure increased to 75 percent of mentally ill aged in nursing homes.[19]

Mental illness is more prevalent in the elderly than in younger adults. An estimated 15 to 25 percent of older persons have significant mental health problems. Psychosis increases after age 65 and even more so beyond age 75. Twenty-five percent of all reported suicides in this country are committed by elderly persons. The chronic health problems that afflict 86 percent of the aged and the financial difficulties faced by many clearly contribute to increasing stress. The stresses affecting the mental health of the elderly are not unique, but they are multiple and pervasive.[20]

The National Institute of Mental Health's evaluation of aging programs indicates that despite the high rates of mental disorder, treatment statistics show that the elderly receive less care than younger adults and their rate of care per 100,000 elderly population is dropping in contrast to the rising care of other adults. Only 4 percent of patients seen at public outpatient mental health clinics and 2 percent of those seen in private psychiatric care are elderly.[21]

In addition, a growing trend in recent years has been to transfer older patients out of costly state mental hospitals into less expensive boarding homes. Very often, these homes lack adequate medical, nursing, social, and psychiatric care. Residents of these facilities are not included in epidemiologic studies of the prevalence of mental disorders among the elderly, which base their conclusions on data from mental hospitals and community mental health centers. The rate of mental illness among the old, therefore, is vastly underestimated.[22]

Despite the magnitude of the problems, and the ever-increasing costs resulting from lack of effective action, appropriate policies and adequate financial support are still not forthcoming.

Less than 2 percent of medicare dollars go into mental health coverage for elderly and disabled beneficiaries. And only slightly over one-tenth of 1 percent of these dollars reimburse community mental health centers for both inpatient and ambulatory care.[23] The medicaid program places emphasis on institutional care; outpatient services are limited. Title XX coverage of social support services relevant to mental health care are also most inadequate. Thus, the entitlement programs often result in unnecessary hospitalization and inappropriate care. Federal support for research and training relevant to addressing mental health problems of the elderly is disproportionately low for the size of the older population and the magnitude of its problems.[24]

Ageism, the attitude that old people inevitably decline mentally and therefore require institutionalization, is held not only by the public but also by medical practitioners, which often leads psychiatrists and other mental health professionals to keep their contacts with old people to a minimum. Avoidance of facing their own aging and death is combined with a belief that emotional problems of aging are simply a self-fulfilling prophecy.[25]

Our policy toward mental health benefits does little to help the old person stay out of the institution. Under medicare, reimbursement for mental health care is even less generous than for physical illness and provides little for outpatient or private psychiatric care; third-party payments, such as medicaid and SSI favor inpatient hospitalization. Nursing homes have become profitable businesses as the federal government pays the owners for each resident, with little care given to the needs and concerns of the aged individual.

The Community Mental Health Centers Act was passed in 1963, in the belief that much long-term hospitalization could be avoided by providing comprehensive care for the mentally ill in the community. Although a number of studies have shown that a majority of geriatric patients do not need long-term hospitalization, the elderly mentally ill are not receiving their representative share of outpatient psychiatric services. Poor economic provisions contribute to this underutilization of care, yet there is evidence that even when coverage is adequate, older persons do not make use of outpatient treatment centers.

Many times CMHCs are located inconveniently in relationship to where the elderly person lives, and transportation may be nonexistent. Some elderly are unable to leave their homes for physical reasons or are afraid to, as many centers are located in high-crime areas. Since health treatment varies in accordance with the social status of the patient—with upper-class patients receiving psychological treatment and the lower-class patients receiving custodial care—the higher proportion of elderly mental patients are working class, and therefore their treatment is also influenced by this factor. In addition, for less-educated and working-class people, there is a stigma attached to receiving mental health services. Targeted efforts not only must be made to reach the elderly with regard to community mental health, but efforts are needed to combine mental health services with a wide range of services, (medical, recreational) so that they become less stigmatized.

The present trend in this country regarding mental illness is toward deinstitutionalization, although adequate alternatives for thousands of unreleased mental patients do not exist. The plight of the elderly ex-mental patient is most difficult, since many have not learned to function outside the hospital setting and are not eligible for job training. On leaving the hospital setting, most are faced with the same isolation, dependency, and lack of treatment they experienced in the hospital.[26]

The President's Commission on Mental Health

In 1977 a presidential commission on mental health was established by executive order with the following mandate: to review the mental health needs of the nation as a whole and to make recommendations to the president as to how the nation might best meet these needs. Special task panels made up of the nation's foremost authorities in mental health were formed to address areas of specialized need.[27]

The panels selected seven major options to reduce the unnecessary and costly dependency of the elderly of the future. They have made use of what already exists legislatively and have built on existing legislation and institutions: the National Institute of Mental Health (NIMH), the National Institute of Aging (NIA), the Social Security Administration (SSA), and the Administration on Aging (AOA). In their report they state:

> These efforts, if adopted, will contribute to the welfare of children who need a humanistic vision of their grandparents and of the later years and who will profit from new knowledge gained through our understanding of the great integrative systems of the body as they change with time and in relationship to age. The traits of a gifted type of adaptation and a wondrous type of survival seen among older people have application to children.

1. Outreach: The problem of accessibility can be ameliorated using an outreach approach, with a coordinator integrating the various services available within the community.

2. Home Care: Home care must become an essential component of the continuum of mental and physical health care of the elderly.

3. Medicare: The discriminatory treatment of mental health services under the provisions of Medicare must be reformed to reduce expensive institutionalization which results from the way current legislation is written.

4. Geriatric Medicine: Geriatric training must become a part of the mainstream of knowledge in preparing doctors, nurses, social workers and psychologists.

5. Research: There must be a major national effort to promote and support accelerated research on the single most terrifying mental health problem of the elderly—organic brain diseases.

6. Allocation of Resources: Resources within the Department of Health, Education and Welfare (HEW) especially in NIMH and NIA, must be allocated in a realistic way as they bear on different age groups.

7. Revitalization of AOA: The execution of all of these options will be heavily dependent upon the effective, revitalized leadership of the specific office created by Congress to be a visible and strong advocate for older Americans—the Administration on Aging.[28]

In September 1977, the "Secretary's Committee on Mental Health and Illness of the Elderly," established by Congress in 1975, reported the results of its study and made a series of recommendations to the secretary of Health, Education and Welfare designed to provide a basic framework for the development of an informed national policy to address the mental health needs of the nation's elderly.

In presenting its recommendations, the committee focused on six major areas of concern: prevention, services, training, research, minorities, and mechanisms for implementation. Although they have been separated for clarity of presentation, all six areas are interrelated.

Prevention

The following eight recommendations were made:

1. Effective systems for teaching the elderly cope with the aging process must be developed. Expanded support should be given to exploring and applying effective strategies for disseminating this knowledge thorugh the media, education institutions, health care providers, senior citizen groups, and other community organizations.

2. Programs that provide the elderly with the opportunity for new and/or continued community roles and activities should receive increased emphasis and support.

3. Increased support should be given to the development, dissemination and expansion of effective models of preretirement and postretirement

education programs, in cooperation with industry, unions, colleges, universities and senior citizens and voluntary organizations.

4. A major program of public education should be developed to combat prejudice toward the old to improve the image of the aging experience in the eyes of the general public.

5. To help provide appropriate services and avoid unwarranted institutionalization, a nationwide system of Comprehensive Geriatric Assessment Units should be created within existing community programs to serve as assessment, assignment, treatment and coordinating centers on an area-wide basis.

6. Crisis intervention programs at the community level should be developed and expanded to provide services for the elderly who are at high risk of developing mental illness.

7. A comprehensive, long-term social support system should be developed in each community for elderly persons who are chronically ill, socially isolated, and/or frail which can provide, on a sustained basis, those services needed to promote and maintain maximum levels of functioning. Existing agencies and organizations should be used to the fullest extent possible, while new models must be designed and tested to ensure that present gaps in services are closed.

8. The most vulnerable groups of the community dwelling elderly should be entitled to special assistance in planning for and access to the services they need: the deinstitutionalized chronically mental ill and those with severely reduced physical and emotional capacities due to extreme old age. Federal support should be given to developing and testing models for sustained community agency responsibility for regularly monitoring and assuring needed services for these high-risk elderly.[29]

Services

The commission recognized that given that at least 15 percent of America's 23 million elderly suffer from significant emotional and/or mental disorders, a national policy needs to be developed to provide a system of mental health services specifically geared to this population. The elderly mentally ill require a full range of mental health services to which they can have ready access. What exists currently, however, are only isolated and fragmented pieces of such a system. Even where services are available, access to these services is hampered by such obstacles as limited reimbursements (Titles XVIII and XIX of the Social Security Act) and inadequacies in current funding mechanisms (Title XX and the Health Revenue Sharing Act, as it related to community mental health centers). Underlying the subsequent specific recommendations are three critical principles which related to the characteristics of the population under consideration:

1. The health and mental health care needs of older persons are interdependent and, thus, the mental health needs of the elderly are best served when they are addressed as part of their basic health care requirements.

2. Elderly persons are responsive to appropriate treatment services geared to individual need. The variability of the health care requirements of the older population—and the changing needs of the individual over time—requires that a full range of mental health services, from ambulatory to full inpatient hospital care, be readily available.

3. Effective linkages are essential between social support services and general health and mental health delivery systems to respond to the interrelated nature of older person's needs.

One of the glaring outcomes of the absence of a policy has been the plight of the deinstitutionalized elderly, where the failure to address comprehensiveness has resulted in the failure to develop sufficient alternatives to institutionalization. The failure to provide continuity of care has resulted in dramatic and all too frequent failures in the transition from institution to community care.

To operationalize all these principles, the committee made the following recommendations:

1. In order to improve the availability and accessibility of mental health care for elderly persons, coverage for mental health services must be provided on an equal basis with coverage for physical health care services, for both acute and chronic illnesses. In existing third-party payment programs, current inequities in coverage for mental health care services must be redressed making mental health care services as accessible as physical health care services, for both acute and chronic illnesses.

2. A national policy to ensure the availability of a full range of mental health services for the elderly, ranging from ambulatory to home health, congregate living, day and/or night care, transitional care, half-way houses, foster homes, rehabilitation services, and specialized inpatient services need to be developed.

3. In order to provide quality mental health services to the elderly, staff of health and mental health facilities providing specialized services to the elderly must have specific expertise and training in geriatric mental health care. Regulations governing third-party payments to such facilities as community mental health centers or other comprehensive mental health program, public or private mental hospitals, or university-operated or affiliated teaching hospitals should require that these institutions demonstrate adequate staff training as a condition of provider eligibility.

4. Staff development and inservice training costs should be an allowable item for Medicare and Medicaid reimbursement up to five percent of total service delivery costs.

5. In long-term care facilities, mental health services should be regularly provided to all patients having significant mental disorders, either directly by the facility or by an outside agency by written agreement.

6. A focal point should be designated at the State level to ensure that the mental health needs of the elderly are being and will be met through careful assessment coordination and planning of state-wide health, mental health and social services.[30]

Research

Subsequent chapters of the report dealt with recommendations to spearhead an expanded national research program on the causes, treatment, and prevention of senile dementia, depression, and acute organic brain syndrome and to establish a national data base on the epidemiology and demography of mental disorders. Psychopharmacological researchers should investigate differential responsiveness to drugs, and increased research emphasis should be devoted to the prevention of the major crises of later life as well as toward an understanding as to the causes, effects, and ways to eliminate prejudicial attitudes toward the elderly.[31]

Training

The committee recommends that a national training effort to develop faculty with expertise in geriatric mental health in the major mental health, health, and social service disciplines be initiated to enhance the geriatric mental health knowledge and skill of existing service providers in the mental health, health, and social service fields. Also, federal efforts should be made to support the development and inclusion of geriatric mental health in the core curriculum and basic training of incoming personnel in all health, mental health, and social service disciplines to be expanded. The committee further urges that a national training effort be supported to develop a cadre of specialists in geriatric mental health and that comprehensive, multidisciplinary training centers for mental health of the aging be created and supported on a regional basis. These centers should be affiliated with appropriate institutions having extensive research and service programs. Content in mental health and aging should be included as a required component of continuing education in programs related to licensure, relicensure, certification, and recertification of health and mental health professionals.[32]

Minorities

Federally funded research and demonstration projects should be established at selected sites throughout the country to explore methods for better serving the mental health needs of elderly minority group members and to conduct research on specific minority-aging issues. The development of strategies for ensuring better access to services for the elderly-minority-group members should be pursued by all federal agencies. Data-collection systems in all federal programs serving the elderly should include provision for reporting of age (by subcategories), sex, race, and ethnic origin. The nationwide training program in mental health and illness of the elderly, recommended by the committee, should make a substantial effort to develop specialized training for serving minorities. In addition, grants-in-aid, scholarships, and fellowship programs should be offered to stimulate minority participation in training for geriatric mental health research, service, and education. Advisory groups and other bodies responsible for evaluating and initiating public programs serving minority elderly should include representation by minority specialists in the aging and mental health fields.[33]

A number of steps to implement these recommendations were outlined that addressed funding, planning, and changes in legislation and asked for the establishment of a "National Commission on Mental Health and Illness of the Elderly" to give special attention to the quality and comparability of statistical data on the aged (for example, their health, mental health, and social status and needs, and types and costs of health and mental health services utilized) that are now collected by each of the federal programs concerned with the general health and mental health needs of the aging population.[34]

At this point, the report on mental health and the elderly, with its urgent recommendations for action, has been submitted to HEW as required by law and awaits its fate as to implementation.

Hospice

At St. Christopher's outside of London, a separate hospital for the care of the dying was founded in the 1950s that came to be called a *hospice*, a term that was used originally to refer to a way-station for travellers. The emphasis has been and is on care for the dying, and schedules are designed to fit the needs of the individual patient and not the institution. The key principle is reduction of pain—physical, emotional, and psychological. It also includes the members of an individual's family in the care efforts and attempts to create a humane environment for everybody involved in the care of the dying person.

In Branford, Connecticut, the first American hospice was developed in 1976. It offers a program for the terminally ill that incorporates the principles of a comprehensive, coordinated program of home care and inpatient care. Particular medical expertise in oncology, in pain control, the management of nausea and other symptoms, maintenance of alertness and mood are stressed. Pharmacological consultation and expert nursing care are given, but, in addition, nurses are specifically trained and given the time to attend to the needs of the patient and the family. Social work, psychiatric consultation, clergy services, and volunteer activities are offered to support patients and families and to include them in an ongoing living process designed to maximize their valuable contribution and participation. In the process of dying and bereavement, it is vital that relationships are lived out and concluded as productively as possible, and families are included as important members of the hospice team, whether the patient is at home or in the inpatient facility.

This emphasis means that the patient and family are involved in both teaching the staff about their needs, and in decision making regarding their treatment. Hospice assists the patient and family to maintain their own lifestyle and a sense of their own responsibility while receiving supportive services.

One of the supportive services in operation is the hospice volunteer program. Volunteers, well oriented to the hospice program, are an integral part of the care-giving service, fulfilling a wide variety of needed tasks, including patient care, family support, and assistance to the staff in planning and community education.

Another aspect of the program is in the field of research and program evaluation. Although some research has focused on the terminally ill, this population has never been observed in a comparative controlled environment such as a hospice will provide. Present research has documented the physical and psychological trauma experienced by the dying and given valuable insights into their special needs. Since hospice offers a situation where these needs are known and generally met, research can concentrate on comparative modes of care. A health care system does not effectively work in isolation. If it is to be most useful to the person in need, it must be integrated into the total fabric of the health care system of the community.

The care that patients will receive in the hospice, although highly personal and specialized, will cost appreciably less than services in an acute-care hospital. Care in the hospice is expected to cost approximately 40 percent less per day than general hospitals. In addition, the home-care program enables the patient to remain home for an extended period, shortening the patient's stay in the facility and further reducing the cost of care.

Although the hospice movement has crossed the Atlantic into Canada and the United States, it is still in a fledgling state, although HEW is interested in promoting the idea. For instance, two Massachusetts hospice programs have ben chosen by HEW's Health Care Financing Administration (HCFA) as sites for demonstration and evaluation projects. The programs will be developed under medicare and medicaid waivers. The American Cancer Society is funding another project to learn more about terminal care for cancer patients.

The Palliative Care Service at the University of Massachusetts Medical Center in Worcester (in cooperation with the Visiting Nurses Association) and the Hospice of the Good Shepard in Newton were chosen in Massachusetts. Two other demonstration projects in New England will take place at the VNA Consortium in Burlington, Vermont, and the Hospice of Branford, Connecticut, the first such program in the United States. Based on the results of demonstrations and evaluation studies, we may expect that further impetus will be given to the development of hospices as part of general hospitals, such as oncology units, as well as in separate facilities, under religious and secular auspices.

Major Issues and Recommendations

Despite all the money funneled into health care, major elderly physical and mental health needs are not being met. As the elderly population grows, the problem of meeting those needs will also grow. Restructuring the health industry would be not just a means for controlling costs but also a means for developing a more comprehensive, efficient, and national system to accommodate those unmet needs.

A restructured system should include such components as: (1) adequate supervised residential facilities for those who lack families, but wish to live in their communities; (2) a range of facilities alternative to the hospital and nursing home, including a system of home care; and (3) innovative and compassionate ways of caring for the terminally ill, outside the hospital and nursing home, such as in hospices. Chronic illness, physical, developmental, or emotional disability or impairment and the problems of advancing age require a comprehensive approach involving a wide range of community services and/or institutional facilities. The continuum of care must include, but not be limited to, acute hospitals, chronic-care hospitals, rehabilitation centers, nursing homes, rest homes, hospices, respite homes, developmental centers, day centers, group homes, and individual homes.

Basic social services are needed to enable persons with chronic conditions who would prefer to live in their own homes to do so. This will require such services as home-health care, homemaker and shopping assistance, handymen and chore services, meals on wheels, telephone assurance, transportation and escort services, in addition to emergency "lifeline systems" and backup services. There also must be recreation, nutrition, referral, legal and mental health and, particularly, dental services.

Comprehensive health care matched to the needs of the individual should be available. A long-term-care system requires a range of care not currently available for the chronically ill and disabled. Short- and long-term health and social care at home and institutions should be available so that the elderly and disabled can return to and/or retain the highest level of independent functioning.

However, if needed, new services are to be promoted, the rate of expansion of the totally medically oriented health industry is going to have to be controlled. Despite government efforts to control costs by regulating the health industry, little success has been achieved. Medical spending continues to rise, much as it has in the past, and the health industry, as presently structured, continues to expand. The powerful economic incentives behind this expansion have so far overwhelmed the regulatory effort.

Since the larger part of the billings of the industry are reimbursed on a cost-plus basis, experiments have been undertaken to pay hospitals on the basis of prospectively approved budgets. But the results are still inconclusive, although some states with such experimental programs have claimed to have achieved significant savings.

The 1972 social security amendments established professional standards review organizations (PSROs) to assure that the services financed by programs like medicare were medically necessary (thus remedying the problem of overutilization of costly hospitals and nursing homes), professionally acceptable, and provided most economically. Unfortunately, this peer-view method of regulation is itself costly, and the results are still inconclusive.

The 1974 National Health Planning and Resource Development Act is to control the expansion of the supply of institutions like hospitals and expensive equipment by requiring, at the state level, the certification of the need for more beds or equipment. But here too there is still no conclusive evidence that the program has slowed down the creation of new and unneeded hospital beds or the addition of ever more expensive and underused equipment.

Current government programs are still biased in favor of institutional (nursing-home) care and against home-based services. If an adequate supply of sheltered-living arrangements, congregate housing, homemaker/home-health care and other community-based services were available, an estimated 20 to 40 percent of the present nursing-home population could be cared for in less intensive and less expensive ways.

A cap on the rate of increase in hospital expenditures and physicians' fees is essential. Hospitals consume a far greater share (40 percent) of health expenditures than any other industry component, and they have had cost increases of about 14.0 percent annually for the last decade. Physicians have been increasing their fees at double-digit rates. Such caps should be continued until surplus beds are eliminated, the rate of increase in hospital expenditures brought into line with average economic growth rates, and the rate of increase in physicians' income brought into line with that of nonmedical professionals.

The restructuring of health service delivery should have the effect of expanding the supply of needed services that are less costly alternatives to hospitals and nursing homes. This requires promoting competing forms of care like HMPs, health care centers, small clinics, and ambulatory health care facilities of all kinds. Greater use would also have to be made of paramedical personnel, especially in underserved rural areas. Government support of clinics, staffed, at least in part, by paramedical personnel would help redress the maldistribution of medical resources. For the elderly, health care restructuring would mean better access not only to conventional medical and dental care, but also to a variety of needed nonmedical social services like home-maintenance services, counseling services, and "linkage" services, which connect the elderly with other forms of care.

Blueprint Illustration

This is an illustration how one state detailed a blueprint for what could happen in the next five years in health care of its elderly population. The basic policy emphasis in the component of the plan that concerns the needs of delivery systems for care of the ill elderly is the aggressive development of noninstitutional services, such as home-health care and intermediate-care facilities for the mentally retarded, coupled with restraints on the expansion of chronic-disease hospitals and nursing homes and the phasing out of existing institutional-service settings such as state mental hospitals.

The emphasis is based on studies that indicate that a substantial portion of nursing-home patients, mental hospital residents, and some retarded people could be maintained at home or in other institutional settings if support services were available. Unnecessary institutionalization is unacceptable because it subjects individuals to the loss of privacy, regimentation, medicalization of life, and lack of contacts with the outside world that are unfortunately common in most institutional settings. To ensure that this policy does not result in the reduction of services to the elderly, mentally ill, or retarded, it is essential that any reduction in institutional services be closely tied to the development of noninstitutional services.

The projection of elderly growth is 16 percent. The plan projects a need of additional nursing beds, especially skilled-nursing beds, but the projected need is less than if the beds were to be as heavily relied upon in 1985 as now. Instead, the plan proposes that adequate community-based services, day-care, and congregate housing be developed to provide alternative modes of care for that portion of the elderly who would otherwise require nursing-home care. There is agreement that elderly and chronically ill should have the choice of remaining in the community, with support services, for as long as possible.

The plan suggests that public funding sources are being stretched thin and will be unable to finance the development and expansion of both community-based services and a growth in institutional care. It is assumed that by shifting to community-based services, a most cost-effective long-term-care system would emerge, and that future costs of providing long-term-care services will increase at a slower rate than if reliance is placed on nursing-home and chronic-disease and rehabilitation hospitals.

The success of the proposed policy reorientation will depend ultimately on the commitment of state and federal governments to financing community-based services and to making necessary administrative and regulatory changes. If this commitment is not forthcoming, major changes in the plan will be necessary.

The plan outlines the need for nursing-home beds, reporting that the state is overbedded in chronic-disease hospitals, that there is a substantial need for more skilled-nursing-facility beds, and that most areas are overbedded in intermediate-care facilities.

It asserts that many patients, who are in these facilities, have only minor disabilities and could be maintained in either rest homes or in the community with support services. Rest homes are residential facilities providing room, board, and some personal-care services. They are licensed by the Department of Public Health. There has been no determination of the future need for this kind of facility for the elderly. A special work group of the Long Term Care Subcommittee of the Health Policy Group has been charged with developing specific recommendations on the proper role of rest homes in the long-term-care delivery system.

Toward a National Health Insurance

For many years there has been talk about a national health insurance system in the United States. Whether a version of such a system will appear is still questionable at this writing. Several plans have been advanced by Congress and by presidents of the last forty years, but none has seen the light of day.[36]

It is the contention of many policy designers that any comprehensive system of national health insurance would have to contain minimally these essential elements:

1. comprehensive benefits with universal and mandatory coverage
2. immediate health-budget cap and rate setting in advance for institutional care and physicians' services
3. a patient-oriented physical and mental health care system with majority representation of consumers on policy-making and administrative boards
4. more primary health care providers with a shift in emphasis and resources away from institutionalization and acute-care services to preventive medicine and health maintenance

5. financing by a combination of progressive employer-employee payroll taxes and general revenues
6. competition among providers with profit incentives to lower costs
7. standards for increasing quality and efficiency of physical and mental health care
8. maximum concentration of program administration at the local level with federal and state public authorities limited in size and scope to providing budgets and guidelines.

The Health Care for All Americans Act proposal has the potential to fulfill these immediate short-range objectives. The Health Care Act would retain the medicare program but upgrade its benefits to provide full coverage of inpatient hospital services, physician services, home-health services, X rays, and laboratory tests. There would be no arbitrary nonmedical limits on the number of hospital days or physician visits. Physicians would no longer bill medicare patients but would be paid directly by the insurance plan, thus reducing the paperwork that has become so burdensome for the elderly. Finally, prescription drugs would be added to the list of medicare's covered services.

Eventually, a much more comprehensive health care insurance mechanism will have to be designed that includes mental health and dental health coverage as well. The experiences of such programs, notably in the United Kingdom, West Germany, and the Scandinavian countries, can be drawn on; their best features can be adopted to the American scene and their flaws and deficiencies can be avoided as we move into the twenty-first century. The introduction of a truly comprehensive national health insurance—in contrast to sickness insurance—to cover all persons according to their health needs would both serve to meet the total health needs of older persons and eliminate older persons as a distinct service group.

Partial national health insurance, for example, coverage of catastrophic illness, would have only a limited impact in this direction; it would not eliminate medicare problems and older persons as specialized recipients. Indeed, catastrophic illness provisions might well so inflate health costs by encouraging expensive forms of hospital care to obtain reimbursement that further cutbacks in regular medicare coverage would be demanded, thereby decreasing the actual benefits to the elderly while fueling possible societal resentment against their "special privileges."

In sum, we need a policy that provides a whole array of linked health services, including home-care, day-care, respite-care, foster-care programs, and sheltered and protective services to deal with the differential physical, dental, and mental health needs of older people, paid for through a national insurance system, as is available in many countries of the world. Institutional long-term care can be organized as a social service with an important health-delivery component rather than the reverse, as is now the case. A well developed home-health program does not obviate the need for high-quality institutional care, but a range of options for patients and their families have to be developed rather than just a single all-purpose solution. The federal challenge is to provide adequate inducements to insure the care of the elderly, no matter what types of health-insurance proposals or health care mechanisms are introduced in Congress.

A restructured health care system must include such components as adequate alternative facilities for those who lack families, a range of facilities alternative to the hospital and nursing home, including home care, and innovative and compassionate ways of caring for the terminally ill outside the hospital or nursing home. The use of hospices is a promising beginning and the late federal demonstration project initiated in 1979 is a step in the right direction. Only a well orchestrated system of physical, mental, and emotional care, system, which is financially underwritten by a national-insurance mechanism, will be able to focus also on prevention of illness and disease and assure a healthier, younger population that can meet the vicissitudes of the later years better fortified and better equipped.

To develop better environmental health conditions is another major task in promoting preventive health care for the young and old. The industrialization, mechanization, and commercialization of our country have produced hazards of grave concern to our health and well-being. Among the by-products is pollution of our physical and social environment. An environmental health policy is of no less importance than an adequate health-care-delivery policy. Such a policy should include: enforcement of existing air-pollution codes and establishment of new ones where needed, with penalties of sufficient magnitude to discourage chronic offenders; research programs to produce nonpollutant engines and other technological innovations to reduce pollution; promulgation and enforcement of the highest safety standards for the automobile industry and strict enforcement of laws aimed at the prevention of highway accidents; establishment of plans capable of treating and converting solid wastes and strict control of industrial wastes and hazards with the cost borne by industry; establishment of a national consumer code with laws to protect consumers by insuring truth in advertising, packaging, and labeling of foods and drugs; renunciation of nuclear, biological, chemical, and all weapons of mass destruction, disavowal of war with its intolerable psychological and physical toll on others as well as ourselves.

Our public policies have to demonstrate that our federal, state, and local governments have a full commitment to consumer participation with professional and paraprofessional health personnel, in the planning, policy, and decision-making processes that go into the organization and delivery of health services, so that the philosophical tenets of the World Health

Organization can become the guiding beacon for health care of the old and the young, whites and nonwhites, those who are financially well off and those who do not share in the wealth of the nation: enjoyment of the highest attainable standard of health as one of the fundamental rights of every human being, without distinction of race, religion, political belief or economic and social condition, as a state of complete physical, mental, and social well-being and not merely the absence of disease or infirmity.

In turn, the road toward achieving this goal is predicated on a public policy that provides for a guaranteed, adequate annual income, decent nutrition and housing, a safe social and physical environment characterized by freedom from fear and prejudice and a spirit of cooperative endeavors.

Notes

1. See George L. Maddox, "Self Assessment of Health Status: A Longitudinal Study of Selected Elderly Subjects," *Journal of Chronic Diseases* 17 (1964):449-460; W.J.A. Van den Heuval, *Older People and Their Health: Some Notes on Health Measurement in Gerontology* (Nijmegan: Gerontologisch Centrum, 1974); World Health Organization, Regional Office for Europe, *The Public Health Aspects of the Aging of the Population*. Report of an advisory group, Oslo 28 July-2 August 1958 (Copenhagen, 1959); World Health Organization, Technical Report, ser. 507 (Geneva, 1970); World Health Organization, *Planning and Organization of Geriatric Services*, Technical Report, ser. 548 (Geneva, 1974).

2. Saad Z. Nagi and Bernice King, *Aging and the Organization of Services* (Columbus, Ohio: Ohio State University, 1976); Saad Z. Nagi, *An Epidemiology of Disability among Adults in the United States* (Columbus, Ohio: Ohio State University, 1975).

3. Eric Pfeiffer, M.D., *Alternatives to Institutional Care for Older Americans: Practice and Planning* (Durham, N.C.: Center for the Study of Aging and Human Development, Duke University, 1973).

4. Ibid.

5. U.S. General Accounting Office, *Home Health—The Need for a National Policy to Provide for the Elderly* (Washington, D.C., 30 December 1977); U.S. General Accounting Office, *Returning the Mentally Disabled to the Community: Government Needs to Do More* (Washington, D.C., January 1977).

6. U.S. Department of Health, Education and Welfare, Office of Human Development Services, *Facts about Older Americans*, DHEW Publication (OHDS) 79-20006 (Washington, D.C., 1978).

7. Ibid.

8. U.S. Department of Health, Education and Welfare, Health

Resources Administration, National Center for Health Statistics, *Health—United States—1976-77* (Washington, D.C., 1977).

9. The law enacted by Congress in 1965 governing medicare is Title XVIII of the Social Security Act (42 U.S.C., sec. 1395). The medicare regulations, promulgated by the Social Security Administration, are published in the *Code of Federal Regulations* at 20 C.F.R., sec. 404.

10. The law establishing medicaid is Title XIX of the Social Security Act (42 U.S.C., sec. 1396). The federal regulations that apply to the state operation of medicaid are published in volume 45 of the *Code of Federal Regulations*, sections 246-250. The regulations governing the operation of medicaid within a particular state are issued by that state.

11. Congressional Budget Office, *Long-Term Care for the Elderly and Disabled* (Washington, D.C., February 1977); Congressional Budget Office, *Long-Term Care: Actuarial Cost Estimates* (Washington, D.C., August 1977).

12. Robert L. Kane and Rosalie A. Kane, "Care of the Aged: Old Problems in Need Of New Solutions," *Science* 200 (26 May 1978):910-919.

13. Sylvia Sherwood, ed., *Long-Term Care: A Handbook for Researchers, Planners and Providers* (New York: Spectrum Publications, 1975); U.S., Congress, Senate, Special Committee on Aging, *Developments in Aging: 1977* (Washington, D.C., 1978), parts 1, 2.

14. Statement made at University of Southern California, in connection with deinstitutionalization program of mental patients in California, Spring 1980. Reprinted with permission.

15. U.S., Congress, Special Committee on Aging, Hearings on *Health Care for Older Americans: The Alternatives Issue*, 95th Cong., 1st sess., 16 May 1977; Robert N. Butler, M.D., *Why Survive? Being Old in America* (New York: Harper and Row, 1975).

16. President's Task Force on Aging, *Report on Nutrition* (Washington, D.C., 1970).

17. Administration on Aging, *Amendments to Older Americans Act, 1978* (see chapter 3).

18. National Association of Social Workers, *News*, February 1980. See also: U.S., Congress, House, Select Committee on Aging, *New Perspectives in Health Care for Older Americans*. Report of Subcommittee on Health and Long-Term Care (Washington, D.C., January 1976); Samuel E. Harris et al., *Alternatives to Institutionalization of the Elderly—the State of the Art* (Washington, D.C.: Sam Harris Associates, January 1976); U.S., Congress, Senate, Special Committee on Aging, "Home Health Services in the United States." Paper prepared by Brahna Trager (Washington, D.C., July 1973); U.S. General Accounting Office, *The Well-Being of Older People in Cleveland, Ohio* (Washington, D.C., April 1977).

19. Robert Kahn, "The Mental Health System and the Future Aged,"

in M. Seltzer, J. Corbett, and R. Atchley, eds., *Social Problems of the Aging* (Belmont, Calif.: Wadsworth Publishing, 1978).

20. Gene D. Cohen, "Mental Health and the Elderly" (Paper prepared for the Center for Studies of the Mental Health of the Aging, Rockville, Maryland, 28 February 1977).

21. Robert N. Butler and Myrna Lewis, *Aging and Mental Health* (St. Louis: C.V. Mosby, 1977).

22. Ibid.

23. Gladys Krueger, "Financing of Mental Health Care of the Aged" (Paper prepared under NIMH contract for the Committee on Mental Health and Illness of the Elderly, 1977).

24. Gene D. Cohen, "Mental Health and the Elderly."

25. Robert Kastenbaum, "The Reluctant Therapist," *New Thoughts on Old Age* (New York: Springer, 1964).

26. Bennnett Gurian, *Current and Anticipated Need for Mental Services and Service Facilities to Meet the Mental Health Care Needs of the Elderly* (Paper prepared for the Committee on Mental Health and Illness of the Elderly under contract to the Gerontological Society, 1977); Stanley J. Brody, *A Preventive Mental Health Program for the Elderly* (Paper prepared for the Committee on Mental Health and Illness of the Elderly, 1977).

27. Federal Council on Aging, *Mental Health and the Elderly, Reports of the President's Commission on Mental Health: Task Panels on the Elderly and the Secretary's Committee on the Mental Health and Illness of the Elderly* (Washington, D.C.: U.S. Department of Health, Education and Welfare, 1978).

28. Ibid., pp. 3-4.

29. Ibid., pp. 46-54.

30. Ibid., pp. 53-60.

31. Ibid., pp. 61-70.

32. Ibid., pp. 71-77.

33. Ibid., pp. 78-82.

34. Ibid., p. 91.

35. Sylvia Lack, "Referral: Hospice," In R. Kalish, ed., *The Later Years: Social Applications of Gerontology* (Monterey, Calif.: Brooks Cole Publishing, 1977).

36. The most prominent plans are the Health Care for All Americans Act of 1979: A proposal by the Committee for National Health Insurance in Collaboration with Senator Edward M. Kennedy and the proposal by President Carter, sent to DHEW in 1978.

6 Housing Policy and Programs

Adequate housing facilities are necessary for everyone; however, the basic needs in housing for older people are somewhat different from the needs of a growing younger family. With smaller incomes and poorer health, older people require less room in their homes. Smaller size and efficient arrangements are important considerations along with proximity to and availability of public transportation and access to shopping facilities, recreation, church, and cultural centers so that the older person can remain active in the community. There are two major elements that combine to make housing for older persons an important issue: one of these elements is social, the other is physical. A striking change in American families at the turn of the century has been the shift from a lower extended multigeneration unit to one that generally includes only parents and their children, the so-called nuclear family. The change has been accompanied by reciprocal alteration in the relationship between older persons and their adult children. The physical nature of many modern American homes and apartments is that they are often not appropriate dwelling units for older persons. Adequate housing also means housing units for older persons that they can afford, that meets the special physical needs of the aged, and that is designed to avoid isolation. Since older people are not a homogeneous group, they need a variety of housing types from which to choose, depending on their health, life experience, income expectations, and personality.

We can differentiate at least four major types of living arrangements: (1) people living at home, either in their own household, with family or relatives, with others, or under a boardinghouse or foster-home arrangement; (2) housing units specially constructed for the elderly, either as a part of the general housing development or as a segregated housing facility under public or private auspices; (3) institutional or congregate group-care arrangements, which would include homes for the aged, nursing homes, hospitals, and so on, and (4) retirement residences, centers, or communities. It has been estimated that 69 percent of the elderly live in their own apartments or homes, 25 percent in other people's homes, 21 percent live with relatives, 4 percent with other people, and 4 to 5 percent in institutions. One out of four older persons lives alone. Living alone is not without difficulties. This is true where there is a couple living together or a surviving spouse. For older couples, who have raised families and through them have resolved many of their differences, it may come as a shock to realize how irritating these differences can become when only two people are involved. Living with one's children may have satisfactions, but it also has its problems if the arrangement is an involuntary one. Generations do not easily adjust to one another, especially when over a span of years their roles are now reversed. When the third generation arrives, many of the difficulties in the child-rearing process may be reactivated; it is not easy for a parent who has reared one generation to refrain from imposing lessons on the next generation. Many older people who live in their own homes often find it quite difficult to maintain them.

Many of the aged living alone live in rooming houses, usually in one of the blighted sections of the city and/or usually shunted off from contact with others. Their sense of isolation and aloneness is aggravated by the problem of living alone in rooming houses that are sometimes maintained by absentee landlords. It has been recognized that for older people to live alone successfully and in dignity, it is essential to have a battery of health and social services that are easily accessible to them. Some of these include home-health care and assistance, friendly visiting, homemaker and chore services, home-delivered meals (sometimes called meals-on-wheels service), transport, and information services so that the older person is enabled to function, if physically and mentally possible, in his own home.

Unfortunately, these services are not found in all parts of the country, and very few of these services are well coordinated even in those communities that have them. They are a great help in making life easier and more comfortable for those whose physical conditions make it difficult or impossible to care completely for themselves. Older people living alone need a battery of professional and paraprofessional services such as visiting nurses, social workers, health aides, home makers, and others.

Some Facts about Living Arrangements

Elderly persons headed 14.8 million or 20 percent of all households in 1976. About 82 percent of elderly family heads owned their home and eighteen percent rented. Among elderly persons living alone, 59 percent owned their home and 41 percent rented. The median value of housing units owned by elderly persons was $25,300, compared to $34,000 for homes owned by younger adults. For black elderly owners, the median home value was $16,200; for Spanish, $19,600. One-sixth (16 percent) of elderly persons in rental housing resided in public housing or government-subsidized private housing. About 4 percent or approximately 1 million older people lived in institutions of all kinds at any one time in 1977. Most older persons lived in a family setting. In the noninstitutional population, the numbers of older men and older women living in a family setting were about the same (7.6

million men, 7.5 million women), but since there are many more older women than older men (146 per 100), the proportion of older men in family settings was 83 percent and of women, 58 percent. About one-third of all older persons (7.0 million—1.6 million men and 5.5 million women) lived alone or with nonrelatives (42 percent of all older women but only 17 percent of all older men). Within the older population the proportion living in family settings decreases rapidly with advancing age.[1]

Income and Housing

It has been assumed that income is a significant factor in the adequacy of housing. How do older people fare in this regard? Table 6-1 compares the number and percentage of older people living in owner-occupied housing units of all incomes and those below the poverty level.

The traditional rule of thumb makes 25 percent of one's current income the "proper" amount to spend on housing. In fact, in 1976, 53 percent of

Table 6-1
Percentage of Elderly Living in Owner-Occupied Housing Units, Living Arrangement, Age, and Poverty Status (1976)

Living Arrangement and Age	All Incomes		Below Poverty Level	
	Number (thousands)	Percent in Owner-Occupied Units	Number (thousands)	Percent in Owner-Occupied Units
Persons in Households	22,100	74.8	3,313	59.6
65-71	10,838	77.3	1,372	63.0
72+	11,262	72.4	1,942	57.1
Family Head	8,128	82.3	725	70.2
65-71	4,316	84.2	355	73.5
72+	3,813	80.1	370	67.0
Living with Relatives	7,100	81.3	560	64.3
65-71	3,748	82.5	282	72.3
72+	3,351	79.9	278	55.8
Living with Nonrealtive	390	67.7	122	64.8
65-71	190	62.1	60	60.0
72+	200	73.0	62	69.4
Living Alone	6,482	58.8	1,906	53.8
65-71	2,585	59.3	675	53.9
72+	3,898	58.5	1,231	53.9

Source: U.S. Bureau of the Census, "Characteristics of the Population below the Poverty Level, 1976," *Current Population Reports*, ser. P-60, no. 115 (Washington, D.C., July 1978).

all those who rented spent under 25 percent of income on their living accom-modations. Among the elderly, however, almost 65 percent of renters and 23 percent of homeowners paid 25 percent or more. For all the elderly, regardless of whether they rent or own, the proportion paying a fourth or more of their incomes for housing was 35 percent.

Eighty percent of all U.S. households are estimated to be able to find unflawed, uncrowded living accommodations for 25 percent or less of their incomes. For 30 percent of income, 84 percent can get adequate housing. But the picture for the elderly is different. Barely 59 percent of elderly households can be expected to find adequate housing for 25 per-cent of income, and only 66.5 percent can find adequate housing for 30 percent of income. Only half of elderly renters can afford adequate hous-ing for 25 percent of their incomes. In comparison, nearly three-quarters of all renters (72.8 percent) can afford adequate housing for the same pro-portion of income.

The elderly who own their own homes are also disadvantaged in this sense. For one-quarter of their cash incomes only 62 percent could afford adequate housing if they had to go out to look for it on the market. For the same proportion of income, 84 percent of all households could afford equivalent housing.

Whether the elderly rent or own, unflawed, uncrowded housing would cost them a much larger proportion of their incomes than it costs the total population. And that is precisely what we would expect, given the precipitous fall in most people's incomes at age 65. What we might not realize is that adequate housing would cost the elderly more, proportionate to their incomes, than it costs the two minority groups—Hispanics and blacks of all ages.[2]

Rising property taxes and home-maintenance costs require that older people spend an increasing amount of their income to keep the residence going. For many people, the decision is simple and obvious: They move to smaller, less expensive, and less physically demanding quarters. For others, this is not the answer. Either financial circumstances make it im-possible to obtain appropriate living arrangements, or their attachment to their home is so great that leaving would cause too much disruption.

More than the purely physical attributes they lose, people most miss the familiarity of the old place. As neighbors and neighborhoods change, people lose that sense of the familiar and may feel that it is time to leave. So, while one segment of the elderly population seeks to maintain familiar attachments, another segment is willing and ready to relocate, particularly if the new setting provides them with more of what they need and want in terms of cost, neighborhood, convenience, comfort, and also access to get-ting where they want to go when they want to go there.

Adequacy of Housing

More of the elderly live outside metropolitan areas than the total population. They live in older housing. They more often own the housing they occupy, and over half have paid-up mortages. The physical adequacy of their housing matches almost exactly that of the total population: only about a tenth of these living units are physically deficient. There is, however, a difference in the housing deficiencies of the two groups: The housing of the elderly has a higher rate of plumbing, sewage, and kitchen flaws than all households; it has a lower rate of flaws in maintenance and toilet access.

Another way to estimate how well households live is to estimate how much of their incomes they must spend for adequate housing. We estimate that 42 percent of the elderly (but only 20 percent of the total population) would have to spend over a quarter of their cash incomes to obtain adequate, uncrowded housing in the market.

The probability of the elderly living in inadequate housing depends on: income, sex, and household size (men living alone have a substantial chance of residing in deficient housing), ethnicity (poor Hispanic men who live alone have the highest chance of being ill-housed, whether they own or rent their housing.[3]

Housing Needs and Housing Policy

Older people wish to live independently as long as they can manage in safety and with some degree of comfort, which gives them a sense of belonging. They want to have opportunities to relate to other people and to engage in social interactions with them. In addition to having a sense of environmental mastery, older people need to be psychologically stimulated by color and sound that is well balanced and well coordinated. Often overlooked is their need for mobility, to be able to move around and to be accessible to shopping, churches, service centers, relatives, and friends.

The key in our housing policy should be to provide options for older people to meet their varied needs as they change during their later years. Yet, more than half of all older people have no real freedom of choice and are dependent on often inadequate available housing arrangements. An issue that cuts across a large variety of housing is whether there should be age mixing or age segregation. Rosow examined the influence of varying proportions of aged persons on patterns of friendship and found that friendship patterns varied in direct proportion to the number of the aged peers living nearby. Age homogeneity yielded the larger number of friendships.[4]

Age segregation of older persons appears to run counter to a major American ideal. Nevertheless, research to date, although by no means conclusive, seems to tip the scale in favor of age concentration in that age-homogeneous environments appear to increase the number of friends and the extent of social interaction, to increase morale, and to contribute to a normative system in which the aged are spared competition and possible conflict with the life-styles of younger persons. It must be noted, however, that at present relatively little is known about how age mixing or age concentration affects middle- and upper-income groups and the younger aged. To the extent that the aged are socially or culturally impelled to form a subculture, age segregation, on balance, may be functional. To the extent that negative attitudes toward old age are changing, thereby enabling older Americans to be partners to other age groups, age segregation may become dysfunctional. Economic factors appear to exert more pressure toward age segregation than do stated policies; migration of younger persons from rural areas and from central cities, low-incomes of the aged and a limited desire to move, all are creating age concentrations of older Americans.

Federal Housing Programs for the Elderly

For some years it has been recognized that the private housing market cannot provide enough adequate housing for low-income Americans. The federal government's first major attempt to address this short-coming in the private market was in the 1937 Housing Act. Since then, especially in the last fifteen years, a number of efforts have been made to encourage the production of low-income housing.

There have been some attempts to assist low-income individuals to purchase their own homes. Elderly participation in these federal programs has been slight. Consequently, the major assistance to elderly Americans who cannot afford adequate housing at market prices has been the provision of rental units. The government has offered loans to developers, often at below-market interest rates, guaranteed mortgages for individual dwellings or projects, and made direct subsidies (payments of monies) available to renters and housing authorities.

Public Housing

By far, the largest housing program has been the low-rent public housing program begun in 1937. To date, over 1.2 million rental units have been constructed of which nearly a quarter (270,000) have been specifically designed for the elderly. In addition, many elderly occupy conventional public housing units as a result of their low income. The Department of Housing and Urban Development (HUD) estimates that as much as 44 percent of the public housing in America is occupied by elderly individuals.[5]

This program is administered by public-housing authorities established within communities. These housing authorities are public corporations established under state housing-authority laws. They are responsible for the construction and operation of the low-income-housing buildings. Projects are owned either by private owners or by the public-housing authority itself. In either case, the authority certifies the eligibility of the tenants.

Mortgage Insurance and Interest Subsidies

A number of past programs have encouraged the construction of rental units for low-income individuals by insuring the mortgage. To qualify under the HUD programs, projects had to be HUD approved, and the money had to be obtained from banks and other private investment sources. In essence, HUD guaranteed organizations that lent money to developers of low-income housing projects that their money would be repaid. Because of this guarantee, banks were able to lend money to developers at lower interest rates.

In addition to insuring mortgages, some programs also provided for an interest subsidy to be paid by the government. The practical result of this interest subsidy was to allow developers to borrow money at much lower rates from private investment sources. For example, a bank would lend money to a developer at 7 percent interest. Of this 7 percent interest, the developer would only have to pay 1 percent and the government would pay the other 6 percent. This reduction of interest cost to the developer resulted in reduced rentals charged to the occupants. These programs are universally referred to by the particular section of the housing acts that authorize them.

Section 236. The major vehicle for government assistance in the construction of multifamily housing was the section 236 program. This program was open to both profit and nonprofit sponsors and offered an interest subsidy that could reduce the interest rate to as low as 1 percent. Some 390,000 units were constructed under section 236, but only about 8 percent were specifically designed for the elderly. This program has been suspended because it failed to provide rental units at sufficiently low rents that very-low-income people could afford.

Section 202: The Direct Loan Program. One of the most popular programs promoting the construction of housing specifically for the elderly was under section 202 of the 1959 Housing Act. Unlike interest-subsidy programs, where money was obtained in the private market, section 202 provided direct long-term loans from the government at 3 percent interest to non-profit sponsors of elderly housing. This program was discontinued in 1969 but was reestablished by the 1974 Community Development Act. Although the original legislation permitted long-term loans and the language was carried over unchanged, HUD's policy now is to grant only interim loans for the period of construction. Sponsors must obtain private long-term financing before the construction loan will be granted. In a ten-year period, the program built 45,000 units in 330 projects.

Section 231. Under another section of the 1959 Housing Act, section 231, HUD provided long-term mortgage insurance for any sponsor of elderly housing. Although this program has not been terminated and is still functioning, it has produced very few projects since 1969.[6]

Provision for meals, housekeeping, and personal care for the disabled or frail elderly has been included in 1978, and since that year the governing board of any nonprofit sponsor must have significant representation of community views to assure increased community involvement in the development and implementation of the project.

Section 8. Although the preceding programs were designed to encourage the construction of multifamily housing by profit or nonprofit sponsors, the 1974 Housing and Community Development Act marks a significant departure from past federal housing subsidy programs. Under section 8, HUD is authorized to make housing-assistance payments (rent supplements) to aid low-income families who cannot find "decent and sanitary" housing in the private sector. The responsibility for financing, construction, and managing housing is almost entirely at the local level.

Under the legislation, communities apply directly to HUD and receive block grants of funds to satisfy the needs of their area. Where existing housing is deemed sufficient, the community will request the required amount of rental subsidy funds based on the needs of the low-income population. If additional housing is needed to supplement existing units, HUD solicits bids from private developers and then awards construction contracts. When the housing is completed, qualified low-income tenants will be able to receive payments under section 8 to cover the difference between fair-market rent and 15 to 25 percent of the tenant's adjusted income. The exact amount of payments to each individual or family is determined by a formula that takes into account level of income, number of children, and extent of medical and other unusual expenses. Fair market rents are established for each community by HUD.[7]

Housing for the Rural Elderly

The Department of Agriculture through its Farmers Home Administration (515 Program) and HUD share the responsibility for providing low-income housing to the rural elderly. The 1978 Housing Act added a rural-rehabilitation-assistance title (section 504) to help rural older people.

As an adjunct to government efforts to assist the elderly to remain in their homes, the concept of reverse mortgage annuity has become accepted. Under this concept, older homeowners are able to convert their home equity into income with the guarantee of lifetime tenure in the home. However, appropriate safeguards must be established to protect older homeowners against fradulent loss of both home and equity in reverse-mortgage-annuity transactions.

The 1978 Housing Act

Section 312 also established rehabilitation loans and authorized $245 million for a low-interest-loan program. Low- and moderate-income owners, occupants, and tenants in multifamily housing are eligible. Households with more than 80 percent of local median income may pay more than 3 percent interest. Financial assistance to housing projects to subsidize housing projects that are in financial difficulty has been authorized in the 1978 Housing Act Amendments that have been characterized by their emphasis on stabilizing and revitalizing neighborhoods, in sharp contrast to the urban renewal orientation of the 1960s.[8]

Innovative Living-Arrangement Options

There have been some innovative developments arising from demonstration projects funded by AOA (Administration on Aging). For example, the Gerontological Institute of the Philadelphia Geriatric Center built intermediate housing in Philadelphia that offers residence in nine small row houses in living arrangements that fall between complete independence on the one hand and institutional care on the other. The houses, situated near the Center, were converted into small apartments to accommodate twenty-seven to thirty-six people. Three or four tenants live in each apartment. The rent, set within the context of social security and SSI benefits, includes building maintenance, janitor service, utilities, and heavy cleaning. Tenants bring their own furniture, and other services can be made available from the Center.

In another experimental project, medium- to large-sized houses are used in a similar manner, establishing cooperative living arrangements known as affiliated housing containing groups of elderly unrelated people who agree to share household expenses, duties, and responsibilities in these houses.

Congregate Housing

A separate funding mechanism for the congregate-housing-services program under the 1978 Housing and Community Development Act has been established. Since the program provides shelter along with nutrition, housekeeping, and personal-care assistance for the elderly in public or private nonprofit housing projects, it can enable many older persons to remain in a residential setting and out of nursing homes.[9]

Under the congregate-housing provisions, HUD is authorized to enter into three to five-year contracts with public housing and section 202 (nonprofit) sponsors to provide congregate services.[10] Area agencies are to participate in planning and are required to review and comment on applications. The employment of elders within such projects is encouraged. In March 1978, a bill to assist frail elderly residents in public housing was introduced in the Senate. The Congregate Housing Services Act of 1978 provides funding directly from HUD to local housing authorities for meals, housekeeping assistance, and other services which can assist impaired residents to remain in their homes and avoid unnecessary or premature placement in nursing homes. The act is an outgrowth of Committee on Aging hearings and reports, which found that congregate services were required by growing numbers of older Americans. Although the program had been authorized since 1970, only a handful of projects had been established because of a lack of service funds. In implementing the program, coordination of support services requires special attention. HUD is going to have to cooperate with the Administration on Aging in evaluating the impact of home maintenance, nutrition, transportation, and homemaker and home-health-service programs that enable the elderly to remain in their homes. In addition, HUD will have to emphasize demonstration projects dealing with residential security and reduction of crime and develop new and innovative approaches to these problems.

Increasingly the public is becoming aware of the potential of congregate housing for many persons who need some daily assistance in order to prolong independence. Various organizations, including the Gray Panthers, are sponsoring congregate-housing arrangements and try to qualify for funding under the housing and community development provisions. Congregate housing fulfills basic shelter and service needs; it can fill the gap between institutional and independent living, maintain independence, and mitigate social isolation.[11]

Retirement Communities

Since the 1950s a number of older persons—couples and individuals—moved to retirement communities in the southern and southwestern parts of the country. In a study of residents of four retirement communities it was revealed that morale was significantly higher for men living in retirement communities than for those who lived in regular communities. Residents in neither community appear to have encountered any difficulty in establishing and maintaining friendship ties. Nevertheless, a smaller proportion of residents in retirement communities than of those in age-heterogeneous communities experienced a decline of close friends and expressed dissatisfaction with their new setting. It was concluded that planned retirement communities not only had provided many opportunities for social activities but also support for those who had a commitment to a retirement life-style of leisure orientation. Persons choosing to live in retirement communities were more likely to desire social and recreational activities than were those choosing age-mixed communities.[12]

Most older persons do not wish to live in retirement communities, many cannot afford to do so, and the health of many will not permit it. But the leisure-oriented who possess the health, the money, and the desire seem to find these communities highly satisfactory. One may confidently expect the number of retirement communities to increase.

Mobile-Home Parks

Mobile-home parks seem to be a fact of life today, although it is known that very few people 80 and over live in trailer parks and that many are forced to relocate when their health declines. There has not been a satisfactory empirical evaluation of the trailer park in terms of the quality of life it supports for the elderly person. Substantial questions remain regarding the effect of such problems as the lack of construction standards, uniform safety codes, or the lack of a clearly specified service role of the management. Anecdotal evidence points to the age-segregated, carefully planned, relatively high-cost trailer park in a mild climate being an entirely acceptable living environment for the healthy young-older person. However, a close inquiry into management practices, access to services, and impact on the surrounding community has yet to be made.

Boardinghouses

Boardinghouses and communal living arrangements have grown up spontaneously, expecially in marginal areas of inner cities. Again, informal observation suggests that they serve a real need. Lifelong isolates and psychologically maladjusted people do grow old, and such people seem to constitute some of the clientele of the boardinghouses, and many are found in fairly desolate conditions and circumstances. Examples abound in many poor neighborhoods of inner cities.

Condominiums and Elders

The "city renaissance" has created problems for elders in neighborhoods. Housing costs have gone up—reflecting the competition for housing—and younger, higher-income persons are at an advantage. As a result elderly are being displaced, and the displacement phenomenon has reached alarming proportions in the early 1980s. Reinvestment in neighborhoods must be done in such a way as to discourage speculation and to equalize benefits among all residents. In recent years conversions of rental apartments to condominiums have hit the elderly particularly hard. Most cannot afford to buy the apartments and are displaced in large numbers, facing evictions at short notice. For this reason special protection of the rights of older persons to decent and secure housing takes on more urgent meaning. Benefits in condominiums include equity and relatively stable maintenance costs (certain services are also included in the cost of the unit), but the lack of national standards for consumer protection and disclosure in sales is a serious problem. The Condominium Act of 1978 was designed to deal with these problems; however, it did not pass during the 95th Congress. Minimum national standards for disclosure and consumer protection for purchasers, owners, and tenants in condominium sales and conversions should be established. Standards are particularly needed to deal with unduly long or unreasonable leases on recreational and other condominium-related facilities that were negotiated by the developer prior to transfer of governance to condominium owners. These consumer protections should be extended to those living in mobile-home parks.

Services in Housing

In several communities across the country, provisions have been made to arrange for a network of health, social, and recreational services to maintain older people in their own homes as long as possible and to avoid institutionalization in congregate-care facilities unless absolutely necessary. For example, as of 1972, the Department of Elder Affairs in Massachusetts, in accordance with its policy to find alternatives to unnecessary institutionalization, provides services directly to the elderly population through home-care services. Home care is offered through a series of locally based non-profit organizations called "Home Care Corporations." They plan, develop, and implement home making and chore services, transportation, information and referral, health maintenance, and legal and nutritional services.

Services such as onsite medical care and common dining rooms are relatively expensive, as are social programs that go beyond the one-day-a-week Golden Age Club. Few low- and moderate-cost housing environments are able to afford these without a subsidy, whether by direct contribution by the sponsor or through local agencies. Onsite meals, in particular, are available primarily because they are made mandatory or because local subsidy makes the service financially possible. It is economically desirable to broaden the consumer base for onsite services by including older people in the surrounding community as potential users. This practice has the even greater advantage of providing intermingling between community residents and housing residents. Thus, in the future, one can expect financial incentives to be made available for agencies and housing willing to make the effort to center community services in housing projects for the elderly. An essential element of such services would be their two-way character: community residents coming to the housing for services and the same or different services traveling to the homes of the less mobile people in the neighborhood.

Medical care is a somewhat different proposition. Economic factors, state licensing regulations, and the aversion of some tenants to the sight of relatively sick people in housing have caused most housing to avoid imbedding any medical care into the service package. Tenant need is very strong for a doctor's office on the site, with regular hours by physician and nurse. Housing combined with a physically separate, long-term-care facility has been successful in other situations, although infrequently for moderate cost.[13]

An Illustration

The United South End Settlements in Boston, Massachusetts, initiated a meeting of a number of community, social, and health agencies with the Boston Housing Authority to explore ways of planning a delivery system of supportive human services to be located within a new combined private and public housing development in the South End of Boston. This system would serve the elderly in both the public and private sectors. The initial contacts were made prior to and during the stage of physical planning and construction of the housing units. The Boston Housing Authority worked cooperatively with a number of social agencies, accepting suggestions related to architectural design, special features such as emergency alarm bells, facilities, and space necessary to house the services. The physical arrangements of this combination of public and private housing with high-rise buildings of seven floors and garden-type dwelling units for families and individuals consists of two seven-story buildings known as "Eva Whiting White Homes," which are the properties of the Boston Housing Authority. These buildings are joined by a landscaped terrace on the second floor level and they overlook a central ground level plaza.

Because of the relatively small size of the elderly population and the facilities, several community agencies found it feasible to develop a model of providing comprehensive services. As a result, the Castle Square services project for the elderly came into existence to demonstrate the value of comprehensive community and health services within housing developments that would provide greater accessibility to services for the residents when needed. The resulting proposal of a system of delivery of services was designed for the elderly residents with the following major objectives in mind: to provide coordinated, comprehensive, and continuous supportive service; to show that these services do help to prevent deterioration and prolong independence of the aging; and to develop a model of a service-delivery system that can be adapted and included in the initial planning and design of public and private housing for the elderly in Boston or anywhere else in the country. One indication that at least part of the objectives were being achieved was the fact that in the two-and-a-half years of the project's operation, just a few tenants had left from the public housing sector to move into nursing homes, two to chronic and mental hospitals, and one couple was evicted. Deaths account for all other residents' departures from the Castle Square public-housing project.

Initially a limited number of services were available when the housing units opened for occupancy. The United South End Settlements provided staff to coordinate the project and develop group work and community programs, as well as a recreation program. The Family Service Association of Greater Boston, Department of Services for Older People, provided a full-time social worker on site in addition to a part-time social work assistant and graduate students from the Boston University School of Social Work. The Visiting Nurses Association of Boston assigned one of its nurses on a part-time basis as an initial step in developing the health component; the nurse assigned had served this area of Boston for more than twenty years and had known or cared for many of the residents during that length of time.

Home Medical Services of University Hospital (Boston University School of Medicine) offered a health-screening program for all residents in public housing and for those elderly in private housing participating in other phases of the project program. Approximately 50 percent responded with findings that resulted in further preventive or corrective treatment or continued followup observation. Subsequently, a clinic was set up and is in operation on a one-day-a-week basis, available to all elderly residents in either housing sector. The visiting nurse, social worker, and physician work as a team in prevention and treatment of health problems of elderly persons. Presently, attempts are under way to secure consultant dental and psychiatric services to round out the health unit. Arrangements have been made with a local pharmacist to pick up and deliver medical prescriptions.

The social services component is another significant part of the program. Of the 125 elderly residents in the public housing unit, the social worker maintains approximately 50 percent of residents as an active case load and 10 percent of the 100 residents in the private housing sector. In line with the objectives of the total program, social service assistance includes any supportive service that the resident needs to function better to maintain himself or to help him through a crisis. Services may be casework counseling, a provision of homemakers, working with a newly discovered diabetic toward acceptance of the illness, shopping for groceries for a temporarily ill client. However, the major thrust of social service has proven to be crisis intervention, and most situations contain a health problem, either physical or mental, or both. The visiting nurse provides health care to patients in the project who are a part of her regular case load. She also screens the patients who are to see the doctor and assists him during clinic hours. The social worker, physician, and the nurse work closely together, and there is continual referring and conferring among them.

The "Companions Unlimited Program" of the Women's Education and Industrial Union accepts referrals of residents in need of a "friend" and also provides transportation to pick up and deliver surplus food items to residents twice monthly. A resident council that meets monthly deals with issues of direct concern to the residents such as safety and security, housing comforts, adaptation and integration with the surrounding community, lack of supervision of small children in the area, and problems that arise largely because of living in close proximity with one another.

A community room is open daily under the supervision of an elderly resident affiliated with the Massachusetts Commonwealth Service Corps who is paid a nominal salary by this agency. There, a variety of activities are offered such as health-information programs, nutritional demonstrations, crafts, music, movies, socials, and programs for special occasions that include dinner and parties. These activities are carried on with group leaders, holiday dinners are prepared and served entirely by residents, and continuous attempts are being made to strengthen existing leadership and to develop new leaders.

The role of the coordinator of the project is vital in linking the various services and in monitoring the delivery. She arranges for conferences and meetings between project and community resources and also serves as staff and liason person to the policy board.

The policy board, composed of board members, executives of the participating agencies, and residents meets regularly to review the project, develop guidelines, and evaluate its operation.

Funding of Services

Securing funding for social services within public-housing developments has been a barrier. In the Housing and Urban Development Act of 1970 provisions to pay cost of dining facility and equipment have been made, although funding for food and other services must be found elsewhere, since there is no direct federal subsidy for social services and there are no national guarantees for resources other than income programs. Although Title XX of the Social Security Act pays for a range of social services, these services, if they are offered, vary dramatically from state to state and community to community. Title XX funds are restricted to programs that provide less than three meals per day and that are not designed to meet the full nutritional needs of people. (A full-meals program in housing does not meet this requirement.)

The emphasis of Title III of the Older Americans Act is on planning and development rather than on support of discrete social services. Its programatic concentration is on needs of low-income and minority individuals, although state and area agencies can support, within funding limitations, a variety of services in congregate housing. Support is legislatively limited to three years, thus it is primarily model-project support and not a source of funds for ongoing service packages.

Medicaid and medicare pay for some home health and home care; less than 1 percent of funds are used for this, but its major emphasis is institutional provision. Block grants via general revenue sharing (Title I of the Community Development Act of 1974) make some funding available for social services. Title I can pay for nonfederal share of grant-in-aid programs. Revenue sharing however is used only to a limited extent for meeting the needs of older people. There is an absence of expressed congressional intent to support social services through revenue sharing. For these reasons, policy should be directed toward creating a categorical-support program that includes an integrated-services component for elderly housing.

Mobility and Transportation

Getting around in safety is a major concern to older people in rural and urban communities. The crimes of force to which elderly are most vulnerable appear to be street crimes—particularly the purse snatch directed toward women and burglary. Although statistics generally reveal that older persons are not victimized by criminal assault against person as frequently as are young males, for example, the special vulnerability of elderly to assault lies in the fact that the impact on them is much more traumatic physically, financially, and psychologically than on younger age groups.

A statistical picture of the incidence of crimes of force on elderly in Los Angeles is revealed by a recent U.S. Census Bureau survey. Of those surveyed who were over 65 years of age, 1 in 56 seniors had suffered a theft (burglary or auto theft); 1 in 73 had been assaulted; 1 in 188 was a victim of purse snatch; 1 in 204 was a victim of robbery; and 1 in 440 was a victim of attempted robbery. In working with seniors, the California attorney general's office crime-prevention unit has developed methods of prevention to minimize the likelihood of victimization by these crimes.[14] Older persons are also trained in techniques of avoiding assault, including when and where to walk, carrying whistles or sirens for deterrence, and the use of the buddy system. Giving emphasis to the positive aspect of prevention efforts minimizes the pervasive climate of fear among older people, who often fear crimes of personal violence considerably out of proportion to the actual likelihood of incidence. Walking is still the most important mechanism for older people to get around.

Relatively well older people report the length of an average daily walk to be about fifteen to twenty minutes. Around two-thirds of them experience no difficulty in walking one-mile. Thus, facilities located within 4 to 6 blocks will be accessible to the great majority of older people, although carrying heavy bundles or making the walk in bad weather will cause problems.

Problems of Transportation

Transportation is a mediator between the person and much of the environment. It determines whether the community is a useless shell or a dynamic social system. Housing, medical, financial, and recreational services for older people are useful only to the extent that transportation is available and useable for the people who need and want the services. Informal social contacts with family members and friends are possible only if access to these persons is available.

Lack of appropriate transportation constricts the life-space of any person, limits his or her capacity for self-maintenance, restricts his or her activities and contacts with other people and may contribute to disengagement or alienation from society. Adequate transportation is not only humane to the older person, it is of economic value to society in that it supports the individual's capacity for independent living and thus assists in postponing or obviating institutional care altogether.

The transportation problem stems from four main factors: (1) many old people cannot afford the cost of transportation; (2) many live in areas that are poorly served by public transit; (3) many older people have difficulty using the public-transportation system; (4) the American transportation system is based on use of the private auto. These factors are interrelated.

Even if older people have enough money to use public transit, services are usually only minimally available in the areas where they live. The rural and suburban elderly are often totally without public transportation; the private auto rules supreme outside the central cities. Within cities, the public-transit system is geared to the rush-hour needs of commuters not to old residents and often is not equipped to accommodate the special needs of older persons.

The root of the problem is the dominance of the private automobile. The car influences land-use and zoning patterns, and highway construction absorbs all but a small fraction of public transportation funds. Even light signals, traffic markings, street signs, and other pedestrian helps are geared toward the smooth flow of automobile traffic—one reason why old people constitute a disproportionate number of pedestrian fatalities. The private auto, with the economic and social changes it has brought about, has destroyed public-transit systems in many cities. When people can afford cars, they stop riding buses, reducing the transit system's income as its operating expenses rise. Fares go up to cover expenses, further discouraging additional riders. Routes are curtailed, quality of service declines, and equipment deteriorates. The poor, the very young, and the old cannot support a transit system caught in this circular dilemma. And all these conditions persist, despite an acknowledged gasoline problem of major proportions.

Furthermore, many older people cannot overcome physical and psychological barriers to the use of public-transit systems. To ride buses and subways requires a high degree of speed, mental agility, and quick reactions. Printed schedules are often largely incomprehensible. It is frequently impossible to obtain information over the telephone from the local bus company. Transportation difficulties are getting worse. The energy crisis, and the subsequent steep increase in gasoline prices, have made it still more difficult for that minority of older people who have driver's licenses to operate automobiles. The process of decline in public transportation systems in both large and small communities is speeding up. The outward thrust of suburban development intensifies everyone's reliance on the private automobile to the detriment of energy conservation mandated by the energy crisis of the seventies and eighties.

Federal action to improve transportation systems for the elderly has unfolded slowly. The Urban Mass Transportation Administration (UMTA) has spent some $2.5 million for research and demonstration projects for the "transit-deprived" groups; less than half this sum has been devoted to projects specifically designed to serve the elderly and the handicapped. However, UMTA has declined to spend an additional $44 million in research, demonstration, and capital-assistance funds, which Congress appropriated. Another source of federal aid is a provision in the 1974 congressional amendments to the Federal Aid Highway Act of 1973, which earmarks 2 percent of the total $6.1 billion appropriation to finance programs for the elderly and handicapped.[16]

More federal aid is to be welcomed, for state and local authorities have shown some willingness to experiment with new methods of serving the transportation needs of the elderly. The most promising of these experiments go beyond the familiar reduced fare for seniors, provided for in the National Mass Transit Act of 1974. Reduced fares, while helpful, do not deal with inadequacies of the existing transit systems nor do they help older people who live in areas with no transportation at all. Rather, these problems are relieved by transportation systems employing a "demand-responsive" concept, a term for a vehicle that comes to your door when you want it, and takes you where you want to go.

"Dial-A-Ride" and other demand-responsive transit systems for older people have been successful in both urban and rural areas. In Rhode Island, the nonprofit Senior Citizens Transportation Corp. provides 10,000 rides annually with 27 minibuses operating on a statewide basis. A similar service operates in mostly rural Missouri, the state that ranks sixth in the nation in the percentage of residents aged 65 and over. Both the Rhode Island and Missouri systems rely on federal subsidies for capital expenditures and operating expenses.

Other experimental transportation subsystems are adapted to the special needs of particular groups of the elderly. These include transportation cooperatives operated by retirement communities, senior centers, or private groups; subsidized use of taxis and jitneys; off-hours use of school buses; use of government-surplus vehicles; and station wagons and small buses operated by social service agencies for their elderly clients. Since 1979, all new public transit buses purchased with federal assistance have been required to have barrier-free design features for the elderly and handicapped.

These special-purchase systems serve evident needs, but they have their disadvantages as well. Transportation experts note that they are relatively inefficient, with a high cost per unit of service. Some are short-lived. Others are inadequate efforts to solve transportation problems that require a high degree of coordinated planning, broadly based funding, and central control.

Specifically, transportation via mass transit has to be conceived as a social service delivery mechanism with infusion of federal funding to assure better and more reliable service, related to the special physical and emotional needs of older persons.

Major Issues and Recommendations

Since housing constitutes a living environment for people and provides the setting and context for a person's daily encounters and behaviors it takes on special meanings not only as physical shelter but also as a mark of identity. The following seven elements are to be viewed as criteria for determining the degree of adequacy of housing for the elderly: age and ownership of dwelling units; the physical condition of the unit; location with regard to services; proximity to recreational, social, religious, and commercial activities; proximity to relatives and age peers; access to transportation; and safety in the neighborhood and in the dwelling.[17] Major issues relate to these recurrent themes in housing policy: maximization of "choice"; retaining and sustaining independent living; need for personal and social services as an intrinsic part of a housing program; and need for continuing and strong federal involvement in making flexible and reasonable funding mechanisms available. Our housing policy must address these themes and be particularly mindful of the changing needs of a new cohort of older people. Therefore the longitudinal study of changing housing needs as people grow older by HUD (begun in 1978 and scheduled for completion by 1988) is of major significance.

Specifically, the following recommendations need to be acted on now: safeguards against arbitrary eviction in the event of conversion of rental units to condominiums; protection of the rights of purchasers of condominiums in accordance with findings and proposals of the Commissioners on Uniform State Laws; establishment of a state housing finance and development agency with powers and funding to encourage public, commercial, and nonprofit organizational participation; encouragement and development of alternatives, such as group housing, to afford older persons greater choice in living arrangements within the community; development of reverse-mortgage-annuity programs with appropriate safeguards to enable older homeowners to convert home equity into lifelong income; development of comprehensive and coordinated services for elders in HUD-assisted housing and involvement of consumers in HUD housing planning. Minority aged and those residing in rural communities need special attention and preferential treatment in the allocation of federal funding.

In view of the elderly's fear of crime it is essential that comprehensive programs of indemnification of victims of crime with restitution by the offender to the victim or the state, with a prohibition against recovery of damages for injuries sustained by a perpetrator, be established; strict enforcement of criminal laws, improved police and judicial procedures and better correctional and rehabilitation programs must be provided; orientation services and special assistance for elderly and handicapped victims or witnesses to facilitate their appearance in court must be established; emphasis on crime-prevention programs aimed at increasing citizen participation in an effort to reduce crime and improve police-training programs must be increased; personnel of the criminal-justice system must expand law-enforcement training to include segments on communicating with and understanding older persons to enable such personnel to deal effectively with the elderly.

Special training programs must be instituted for housing managers and other types of housing personnel to sensitize them to the differential and changing needs of their aging residents as well as to acquaint them with those services that are available in the community to cope with occurring problems or sudden crises. As adequate transportation is an essential service and must be a part of all programs for the elderly the following action is to be sought: the use of publicly owned or operated passenger vehicles at lowest possible cost during the hours they are not otherwise in use and on weekends for the transportation of elderly persons; standards for reexamination of licensed vehicle operators based not solely on chronological age, but rather on functional age and driving record; the frequency of such reexaminations should be determined without prejudice to older drivers; reduced-rate fares for the elderly on public intrastate transportation; and the development and operation of special mass-transportation subsystems, particularly in rural and suburban areas.

Notes

1. U.S. Department of Health, Education and Welfare, Office of Human Services Development, *Facts about Older Americans*, DHEW Publication (OHDS) 79-20006 (Washington, D.C., 1978).

2. U.S. Department of Housing and Urban Development, *"How Well Are We Housed?" The Elderly* (Washington, D.C.: U.S. Government Printing Office, 1977).

3. Ibid.

4. Irving Rosow, *Social Integration of the Aged* (New York: The Free Press, 1967).

5. U.S., Congress, Senate, Special Committee on Aging, *Hearings on Adequacy of Federal Response to Housing Needs of Older Americans* (Washington, D.C., 1971-1976).

6. U.S. Housing Acts of 1959 (12 U.S.C. 1715 Z-1), as amended, secs. 202, 231, and 236.

7. U.S. Housing and Community Development Act of 1974 (42 U.S.C. 4501), esp. sec. 8.

8. U.S. Housing Act of 1978 (PL 95-557), secs. 312 and 504.

9. Frances M. Carp, "The Concept and Role of Congregate Housing for Older People," *Congregate Housing for Older People*, International Center for Social Gerontology, prepared for the Dept. of Health, Education and Welfare (Washington, D.C., 1977).

10. U.S. Housing Act of 1978; Congregate Housing Services Act: (PL 95-557, Title IV) U.S. Dept. of HUD, Washington, D.C.

11. Wilma T. Donahue et al., *Congregate Housing for Older People, An Urgent Need, A Growing Demand*, U.S. Department of Health, Education and Welfare, Office of Human Development, Administration on Aging (Washington, D.C., 1977).

12. G.L. Bultena and V. Wood, "The American Retirement Community: Bane or Blessing?" *Journal of Gerontology* 24 (1969):209-217.

13. *Developments in Aging*, 1978, Chapter VII and *Appendix*, pp. 255-267, and U.S., 95th Congress, House, 2nd session, Select Committee on Aging, *Hearing on Housing the Elderly: Integration of Health and Social Services* (Washington, D.C., March 1977).

14. U.S. Bureau of the Census, *Current Population Reports*, no. 59, May 1976.

15. Ibid.

16. *Transportation and the Elderly: Problems and Progress*. Hearings before Senate committee (Washington, D.C., 1978).

17. Frances M. Carp, *A Future for the Aged: Residents of Victoria Plaza*, 1966, Austin: Univ. of Texas Press and "Housing and Living Arrangements of Older People" in R. Binstock and E. Shanas, eds., *Handbook of Aging and the Social Sciences* (New York: Van Nostrand Reinhold, 1976), pp. 244-271.

7

Social Service Policy and Programs

There is little agreement in the literature or among the social systems of different countries as to the definition of social services and social supports and what is to be included under these rubrics. Although they have many commonalities, there is much variation in the goals, organization, and content of social services to the aging throughout the world. The White House conferences on aging in 1961 and 1971 defined social services as a flexibly organized system of activities and institutions to help attain satisfying standards of life and health, while helping people develop their full capacities in personal and social relationships. For older persons they are those organized and practical activities that conserve, support, protect, and improve human resources. These programs include: financial assistance, case work, counselling, information and referral, friendly visiting, group activities, and protective services.[1] This is a generally accepted definition based on the collective ideals of common human needs and human-life-span development.

Social Supports and Social Services

The aging process represents a continuum: being old is not being different from the rest of the population. Therefore, the basic needs of older individuals will be more similar to rather than different from other age groups. Granted, the aging process may indicate that certain needs may be more prevalent at some periods of life. For example, the elderly individual, because of declining physical strength, may not be able to get around with the same facility as in the past. However, this need to get from one place to another will probably remain the same, and, as has been pointed out, this need must be met through special access facilities to public transportation or specially developed transportation systems.

Although there is continuity in development, individuals and their cohorts are influenced by the accumulation of events. Thus, people vary from each other as a result of idiosyncratic experiences in their lives, and likewise age groups are influenced by historical events and social and cultural developments such that we can expect that the elderly population in twenty years will be different in significant ways from the elderly population of today. Therefore a variety of programs must exist to respond to individual needs. In addition, programs must change over time in anticipation of the different experiences of successive cohorts of elderly individuals.

Human beings grow, develop, and mature as a result of a combination and interaction of biological, social, cultural, and other environmental factors and to diminish or remove any one is to alter the quality of human existence. In Western society old age is not defined in terms of functional capacities; rather it is defined formally and chronologically. At age 65 one is considered old and is thereafter regarded as if functional capacities had declined. Individuals thus regarded have problems rather than differential needs. We think of these as social problems, which have their source in the social definition of old age, that primarily affect the young-old, those approaching or recently past 65. These are culturally specific problems, affecting only those individuals unfortunate enough to turn 65 in a society that equivocates that age with functional incapacity. These persons must cope with problems like retirement, a social invention of industrialized society. Retirement often brings a drop in income accompanied by a nagging sense of uselessness, born of an awareness of low social worth.

The greatest danger of functioning problems in old age is that the older person's ability to continue living in the community is threatened. The greatest danger of social problems in old age is that the person will come to accept that definition of functional incapacity and low social worth. Both the young-olds and old-olds are thus often in a situation of increased dependence. The dependence might be economic, political, emotional, or expressed in other forms. The point is that this ever-increasing dependency raises an important issue for older persons. On whom shall they depend?

Societies vary in their response to the increased needs of their older members. In sixteenth-century England the aged were licensed to beg on the streets. Beyond this dubious privilege the government offered no assistance to the elderly. They were expected to depend on themselves. In seventeenth-century England a different approach was taken. Families were held legally responsible for the care and support of their older members, just as today parents are responsible for their children. In fact, the most common response of societies to the problem of needy elderly has been to expect, morally if not legally, that children will care for their aged parents. Thus the quality of life in old age has often been related to the ability and willingness of younger family members to allow older members to depend on them.

Maslow suggests that human needs can be arranged in a graduated series on a hierarchy.[2] The levels of the hierarchy are arranged on a line starting with the most basic physiological needs and then running through a continuum of increasing sociocultural needs. The following five levels are outlined by his theory, starting with the most basic and moving onto higher levels: physiological needs (food, shelter, clothing, sex); safety needs (security and stability); belongingness and love needs (identification and affection); esteem needs (prestige and self-respect); and self-actualization needs (development of individual potentials). There are two key assumptions in his theory: first, a lower need must be well on the way to being satisfied before the next higher need can fully emerge. This is related to population heterogenity and the necessity of varied and flexible program response due to varying ability of individuals to meet their own needs. In addition, as society fulfills the basic needs of its older citizens, new needs will surface requiring additional programs. Second, satisfaction of the higher needs brings an individual a sense of worth, dignity, and accomplishment, and therefore the ultimate satisfaction of these needs is necessary if the autonomy and dignity of the elderly in the community are to be maintained.

The effect of social service programs can be to increase the available problem-solving alternatives, thereby maintaining autonomy and dignity. For example, if older people have trouble getting around and need to travel to medical appointments they have several alternatives. They might try to get there on their own, or they might ask a friend or relative for a ride. Or, if the community has a transportation program for the elderly, they could take advantage of this service. The alternatives available for old people who need rides have thus been increased through the provision of a social service.

There is a sociological principle here that is important in understanding the provision of social services to the elderly. It is naive to see any of the programs as exclusively in the interests of the aged. If services were designed and implemented with only the aged in mind, they might expand until all the needs of older Americans were met. There might be, at least theoretically, no limit to the services provided. This is clearly not the case. The funds allocated for elderly social services have real limits. All the services are not available to all those older persons who may require them. Decisions are made as to which services will be made available, where these will be located, and who will be eligible to receive them. But other groups are also served when services are provided to the elderly. Consider the interests of the middle-aged children of older parents. Without governmental services they might be totally responsible for their aging parents. As this middle-aged group is primarily responsible for paying taxes that funds programs for the elderly, we can understand also why there are real limits to the number and quality of services provided.

The interests of those in political office offer another explanation of why some services come into existence while others do not. Politicians need to demonstrate to their constituents that the elderly programs they endorse are meeting their stated goals and are cost efficient. Politicians are therefore likely to align themselves with those programs that can show, relatively quickly, tangible results.[3] If politicians were exclusively concerned with the interests of the elderly, then we would expect that they would also take unpopular stands to protect the needs of the elderly against program cuts. Again, this is often not the case. The tax revolt of the seventies, accompanied by the rapid retreat of many liberal politicians from support of social services, is an illustration of the point. The extent to which politicians will uphold or abandon services for the elderly is a function of electoral assessment at least as much as it is a function of elderly needs assessment.[4]

A third group that has a direct interest in services for the aged are the human service professions, notably social work. Social work is increasingly dependent on government programs for its continued existence. Services to the elderly represent a potential job market for many social workers. A dominant motivating goal in American society for professionals and nonprofessionals alike is "success."[5] Social workers are also influenced by the pursuit of fame and fortune as are doctors, lawyers, bankers, or corporate managers, although to a considerably lesser extent. Therefore we can expect social work's commitment to services for the elderly to be directly related to the actual or potential government funding of these programs: "The very incentive systems that create and sustain their organizational viability—the interest of their members and the pursuit of their trades and professions—precludes them from testing the extent of their power to achieve fundamental changes for the aging."[6]

Social services for the elderly do not exist in isolation. The interests of the aged sometimes coincide and sometimes conflict with the interests of other groups in society. In situations where provision of a service meets the taxpayers need for low cost, the politicians need for demonstrable results, the social worker's need for employment, and the elderly's need for service, we would predict a likelihood that the service might come into existence. Similarly, when the need for the elderly stands alone, we would predict a less vigorous response by the society to that need.

Types of Social Services

We can differentiate three major types of social services: (1) services provided to all older persons as a "social utility," regardless of proven need; (2) supplementary services needed by older persons with temporary problems in their adjustment to becoming older; and (3) special services necessitated by social or personal conditions that are permanent and lasting.

As discussed before, the two supporting legislative pillars sanctioning programs and services to the aged are the Social Security Act of 1935 with its amendments and the Older Americans Act of 1965 and its amendments. Federal provisions of social services to the aged date from the 1962 Amendments of the Social Security Act. In 1975, Title XX of the Social Security

Act, the "Social Service Title," was implemented. Its major stated purpose is to reduce dependency and promote self support for all age groups. This title is geared to segments of the older population who can claim and document financial need. Eligibility is confined to recipients of supplemental-security income (SSI), established in 1974 as a successor to the Old Age Assistance Program. Each state may determine additional populations over 65 who are financially needy and can qualify (see chapter 4). The states are required to provide certain services while others are optional. Overall, there has been a large area of discretion at the state level, with regard to the extent and kinds of services that might be offered.

Mandatory services for the aged (also the blind and disabled) include the following: information and referral without regard to eligibility for assistance; protective services; services to enable persons to remain in or to return to their homes or communities; supportive services that would contribute to a satisfactory and adequate social adjustment of the individual; and services to meet health needs. Optional services that any state might elect to include encompass three broad categories: services to individuals to improve their living arrangements and enhance activities of daily living; services to individuals and groups to improve opportunities for social and community participation; and services to individuals to meet special needs.

By contrast, services provided under the Older Americans Act are universal because they are not based on proven financial need. Efforts are made to channel resources to those communities where minorities, women, and single older persons live; this is because it is assumed the percentage of elderly with money needs is highest in those communities. The Older Americans Act defines social services as follows: health, continuing education, welfare, informational, recreational, homemaker, counseling, or referral services; transportation services where necessary to facilitate access to social services; services designed to encourage and assist older persons to use the facilities and services available to them; services designed to assist older persons to obtain adequate housing; services designed to assist older persons in avoiding institutionalization, including preinstitutionalization evaluation and screening and home-health services; or any other services if such services are necessary for the general welfare of older persons.

As stated, the major distinction in public service provision for the elderly is that some services are universal and some are selective. Services provided under Title XX of the Social Security Act, are selective, means-tested services. Financial need and age (65 and older) are the basic criteria for eligibility for these services. At present, all recipients of SSI, plus an additional percentage of those with incomes under 80 percent of median income, may be eligible for services. (Under Title XX, eligibility criteria may vary with the service.) No firm, comprehensive data (dollars, services, number of recipients) exist as yet with regard to service utilization by older people.

In contrast, services provided by programs under the Older Americans Act are designed to be universal, not means-tested, although a deliberate effort is made to direct provision to communities in which the percentage of elderly "at risk" is highest (minorities, women, single). As much can be said about programs provided for the aged by the voluntary sector, which also tend to be regarded as universal.

In general, funding and extent of coverage of social service is limited and nowhere near adequate for the number needing and wanting them. The major congregate-meals program is designed to serve about 1 percent of the elderly (the target population the program addresses is equal to at least 16 percent of the elderly); it is generally agreed that senior centers are overcrowded and haphazardly placed; reduced-fare programs are heavily utilized but they exist in only about a hundred cities. Often, even where services may be available in the market, costs are prohibitive for the poor, the working class, and some times even the middle class. In contrast, in a number of metropolitan areas, free or reduced-fare (50 percent) transportation on public transport is available to the elderly; and delivered or congregate meals may be free, priced at what the recipient wishes to pay, or offered at very low, below-cost levels.[7]

Declaration of Objectives for Older Americans

The major goals of programs and services to an increasing older population have been summarized in the preamble of Title I of the Older American Act of 1965:

> Sec. 101. The Congress hereby finds and declares that in keeping with the traditional American concept of the inherent dignity of the individual in our democratic society, the older people of our nation are entitled to, and it is the joint and several duty and responsibility of the governments of the United States and of the several states and their political subdivisions to assist our older people to secure equal opportunity to the full and great enjoyment of the following objectives:
>
> 1. An adequate income in retirement in accordance with the American standard of living.
> 2. The best possible physical and mental health which science can make available and without regard to economic status.
> 3. Suitable housing, independently selected, designed and located with reference to special needs and available at costs which older citizens can afford.
> 4. Full restorative services for those who require institutional care.
> 5. Opportunity for employment with no discriminatory personnel practices because of age.
> 6. Retirement in health, honor, and dignity after years of contribution to the economy.

7. Pursuit of meaningful activity within the widest range of civic, cultural, and recreational opportunities.

8. Efficient community services, including access to low-cost transportation, which provide social assistance in a coordinated manner and which are readily available when needed.

9. Immediate benefit from proven research knowledge which can sustain and improve health and happiness.

10. Freedom, independence, and the free exercise of individual initiative in planning and managing their own lives.[8]

Categorization of Services

Based on the locus of service delivery the following categorizations can be differentiated: in-home services, that is, services delivered to persons enabling them to remain living in their homes alone, with their spouse or other family members as part of the community, and out-of-home services provided to older persons residing in institutions.

Virginia Little cites a new terminology which has grown out of studies sponsored by the European Centre for Social Welfare Training and Research: *open care* in the community, encompassing all programs aimed at supporting living in one's home; *closed care* encompassing care in institutions; the term *nonorganized care* is reserved for informal support systems (natural networks) that include families, relative, neighbors, friends, community care takers and irregular volunteers. Open, closed and nonorganized care are found side by side in every society, according to Little.[9]

Open Care

The major types of in-home services are health care support, social support, and access and assistance services. In-home services have three goals: (1) to maintain older persons in the familiar surroundings of their home, in the community or neighborhood for as long as physically and mentally warranted, and thereby avoiding unnecessary and premature institutionalization; (2) to keep older persons close to family, neighborhood, and community ties; and (3) to provide responses to the needs of older persons and their families during various times in their lives, thus assuming greater flexibility in caring for them.[10]

Noninstitutional community services have played a major role in the care of the aged and disabled in Britain and other European countries for a long time. By contrast, in the United States there have been relatively few home-related services to supplement the rapidly expanding institutional services. In Western Europe, existing community services are usually centrally organized and closely tied in with health care. In the United States, community services are more likely to exist under the auspices of special sponsoring groups under governmental or nongovernmental auspices, such as religious or secular organizations.

Each municipality in the United States has special resources and services to benefit the aged and disabled. However, their development has been sporadic, frequently haphazard, often emanating from the specific functions of individual agencies, as interpreted by an agency board and staff, rather than stemming from a broad definition of community needs. This can be said of voluntary as well as public agencies. The latter are set up and function to carry out legislation or regulations authorized by federal, state, or local governments. The following is a brief description of major services in all three categories.

Health Supportive Services

Adult Day-Care Centers. Adult day-care centers are social programs for frail, moderately handicapped, or slightly confused older persons who need care part of the week. Often they live alone and cannot manage by themselves, and by sharing some of the responsibilities for care, the family is able to help the older individual remain independent. Day centers are oriented to rehabilitative, physical, and other types of therapeutic health care. Although day care is relatively new to the United States, it has been utilized in Europe for many years.

Day care began with the passage of the Social Security Act Amendments of 1972, which authorized an experimental program to provide services to individuals eligible to enroll in the supplemental-medical-insurance program established under Part B of Title XVIII of the Social Security Act and meet the standards established by the Secretary of HEW.

Its basic goals are to provide social contacts, enrichment experiences, and to lighten the burden for younger families or for children who must work. Day-care furnishes activities for isolated elderly, some transportation for travel to medical clinics, dentists, and doctors offices, and recreational therapists. A center may also offer health services on-call for people who may need them. The day-care center approach is to insure that people have pleasant surroundings where they can carry on certain activities commensurate with their physical needs, social functions, and conditions.

Home-Health Care. Home-health care programs have increasingly come into their own in the last decade. The Visiting Nurse Association or the Public Health Nurse Service offer care to older persons who are referred to them by hospitals, councils on aging, home-care corporations, area agencies, community centers, multiservice centers, and so on. The staff of the Visiting Nurse Association usually sees older adults in their homes and if needed, they administer medication under the instruction of a physician. Nurses also look for social problems that may exist and notify other community agencies that can supply needed social support. In addition, physical, occupational, and speech therapists may provide services on all on-call basis or they can be included in a coordinated home-health-care program.

Home-health aides are paraprofessionals who provide personal health care assistance, usually working under the supervision of nurses. Their services include interviewing and screening patients to discover unmet needs. Such needs are then brought to the attention of a nurse or physician.

Home Medical Service. Home medical service is another health-support service that sponsors visits to older patients. This service is offered by nurses, occupational therapists, physical therapists, and social workers or physicians who, in many instances, are residents or interns at medical schools affiliated with hospitals. Relatively few communities offer these types of medical services. A notable example is Boston University's Home Medical Service; for over one hundred years it has made this service available, rooted in a conviction that students in medical training should be exposed to the milieu of older patients. Based on this pedagogical concept, a regular service emerged that exists today in Boston's South End.

Nutrition Programs. Nutrition programs are made possible by enactment of Title VII, now part of Title III, of the Older Americans Act, which also provides transportation and social programs. The major focus of this program is to satisfy the nutritional needs of ambulatory persons and to meet social needs by offering congregate meals at a nutrition site. Meals on Wheels is another nutrition project. Meals are served directly in a persons' home. Usually a paid cook or a dietician takes responsibility for food preparation, and volunteers to deliver the meals to the elderly. This program was pioneered in Western Europe and has now found popularity in the United States, although it is by no means offered in every community.

Congregate meal sites established under this program must serve at least one hundred meals daily, five days a week. Individuals 60 and older residing in a project area are eligible for the service and decide for themselves the charge for a meal. No means test is required.

Other congregate-meal services are located in or affiliated with school cafeterias. School cafeterias may prepare food either for service to older persons after the students' lunch hour or to be delivered to other locations and served there. Some states have passed legislation reimbursing any school or nonprofit organization for the expense of serving a meal to the elderly, over a certain cost.

Social-Support Services

Homemaker Services. One of the most widely known social support programs is homemaker services. The program is an important alternative to premature, unnecessary institutionalization. The primary goal is to enable older, or disabled, individuals to remain in their normal environment. Homemakers are usually nonprofessionals or volunteers. Their duties include the personal care of the client, friendly visiting, and home-help jobs, such as cooking, shopping, and house cleaning. Increasingly, a difference is being made between a home maker and a chore service provider who merely does the housework but does not offer personal care.

Both services are usually administered by public or private family and children's agencies, directly, or under contract with a nonprofit or profit-making group. For example, the Upjohn Medical Company has established a large homemaker-service division, and several public and private family agencies subcontract with them. A number of autonomous home maker agencies have emerged and a national organization, the National Council for Homemaker Services, is moving toward establishing professional criteria, accreditation procedures, and training programs.

The distinction between the home-health-aide services and home-maker services is mainly administrative. The health agency and health aides are supervised by public health nurses instead of home-maker supervisors or social workers. The designation of the term "chore services" is an attempt to upgrade domestic work, thereby giving workers more status, better salary, and some fringe benefits.

Counseling Services. Counseling services on an individual or group basis are offered by social agencies, either through departments of public welfare, private family-service organization, social workers, or psychotherapists. The majority of counseling services are agency based, and older persons are expected to take the initiative and go to these agencies. Settings where counseling or case work are offered include privately sponsored family-service agencies, community mental health centers, well-aging clinics, general hospitals, mental health institutions, geriatric day hospitals, adult day-care centers, multiservice centers for older persons, settlement houses, public health and public welfare departments, and other social agencies.

The following five problems that require counseling have been identified in several studies: (1) Problems in individuals adjustment and family relationships. While there were relatively few marital problems (evidenced by the fact that few of their clients were still married), many of the problems concerned relationships between aged parents and their adult children that can be labeled as "intergenerational conflict" and "filial crisis" and problems of isolation and loneliness. (2) Problems of physical illness and medical planning. They were numerically most significant as there was a link between physical illness and emotional breakdown, and physical illness in one of the partners, when they were still married, created heightened anxiety. (3) Acute breakdown and inability to manage their own affairs. These were problems whereby many of the people living alone could no longer fulfill their regular responsibilities and needed assistance, home care, and, at times, protective services. (4) Economic problems, such as financial deprivation as well as problems with a budgeting and shopping. (5) Living and housing problems. Older people found it difficult to adjust to their home and living situation or to an institutional setting.[11]

Outreach counseling services by social service personnel, usually in combination with other health professionals, are still quite rare, although much needed. Outreach service is not to be confused with outpatient services. Outreach programs endeavor to locate the elderly in need of care within the community and facilitate their contact with available caregivers and agencies. Outpatient services are those direct health services that are provided on an ambulatory basis.

Crisis Intervention. According to crisis theory, "a period of upset during crisis may be a potential turning point when the individual's vulnerability to immediate or eventual mental disorder may alter significantly; in a time of crisis there is increased openness to accessibility of the individual that can lead to both adverse and salutary consequences."[12] The outcome of crisis intervention is dependent on a person's constitutional resilience, precrisis adjustment, coping skills engendered by other crises, general helpfulness contained within the social network, and specialized help stemming from a person's understanding of the circumstance of the crisis. Several community agencies provide crisis-intervention services and crisis supports to the elderly who are often beset by physical, emotional, and social crisis that result from problems of poverty, disability, illness, loss of spouse, friends, and so on. Delay in responding often produces far more damaging consequences than if an immediate response had been forthcoming.

Multiservice Centers. A program providing a combination of services is the senior center. The first publicly supported senior center was established in New York City about thirty years ago, and the number expanded gradually until about ten years ago. The expansion of this type of program was accelerated by authorizations of Title V of the Older Americans Act (now part of Title III), which provided funds through the AOA's state programs to communities to assist them in developing center programs and also, since 1976, for construction of facilities. During this same period, public housing for the elderly was designed to include space for center programs for residents of housing developments as well as other older people from the neighboring community.

Voluntary organizations, both sectarian and nonsectarian, have also been active in developing and operating such programs. A directory of senior centers in the United States, published jointly by the AOA and the National Council on Aging, listed 340 such centers in 1966; a more recent directory, published in 1975, listed 5,000, and the number keeps increasing.[13]

Centers vary greatly in the kinds of programs and services offered and in the elaborateness and adequacy of physical settings, but each offers some contact with other elderly people and some links with needed services. Although, for the purpose of the directory, the definition of a senior center is "a program for older people provided in a designated facility open 3 or more days a week," the average center listed offered three or four recreational activities and one or two types of counseling and community services. Among the typical services offered (and the best centers provided at least several of these) are the following: information, referral, and brief direct services; case-work assessment; case-work counseling; service coordination; medical and psychosocial diagnosis; home-health care; financial management; legal services and/or guardianship; transportation and/or escort services; cash for emergencies; volunteers' services; delivered meals.

A senior center seeks to create an atmosphere that acknowledges the value of human life, individually and collectively, and affirms the dignity and self-worth of the older adult. This atmosphere provides for the reaffirmation of creative potential, the power of decision making, the skills of coping and defending, the warmth of caring, sharing, giving, and supporting. The uniqueness of the senior center stems from its total concern for older people and its concern for the total older person. In an atmosphere of wellness it develops strengths and encourages independence while building interdependence and supporting unavoidable dependencies. It works with older persons not for them, enabling and facilitating their decisions and their actions, and in so doing it creates and supports a sense of community that further enables older persons to continue their involvement with and contribution to the larger community.

The philosophy of the senior center is based on the premises that aging is a normal developmental process; that human beings need peers with whom they can interact and who are available as a source of encouragement and support; and that adults have the right to have a voice in determining matters in which they have a vital interest. As such, the center is a major community institution that is geared to maintain good mental health and to prevent breakdown and deterioration of mental, emotional, and social functioning of the older person.[14]

Telephone Reassurance. Telephone reassurance programs offer a significant social and psychological support service. Many communities have started telephone reassurance chains linking theirs to an existing "aging network" agency, such as a council on aging, a senior center, a private organization, or a volunteer group. The goal of this service is to provide a "cue-check" to discover if the person needs assistance or if any emergency has occurred. Persons called on the phone daily also have an opportunity to reach out socially to others.

An adaptation of this program is Life Line, a newly developed emergency alarm system, that was pioneered by Life Line, Inc., the Boston University Gerontology Center and the Hebrew Rehabilitation Center for the Aged in Boston and is now in operation in over 20 communities. A mechanical device is attached to the telephone in an older persons' home. This mechanism enables the person to start an alarm signal, which is activated at a central station. An operator receives the signal and in turn, provides assistance. Life Line also acts as a "psychological reassurance" because the older person knows that next to his or her bedside, via a portable trigger, there is immediate access to an emergency station that can provide help.[15]

Group Work. This service and treatment form has been in use for several decades. Originally performed as a spontaneous recreational activity in centers for the elderly or in golden-age clubs, it has become recognized that group work demands specially trained personnel with special skills. More and more recreation centers, golden-age clubs, day-care centers, family agencies, general and geriatric hospitals, public welfare departments, homes for the aged, and so on have begun to develop specialized group-work services when older people find it difficult to cope with peer and social relationships. Groups are formed with the help of a social group worker, and the group experience of the members is utilized for resocialization purposes. Group workers are attuned to individual needs and work with individuals in the group and also outside the group and, if necessary, make referrals to other community agencies, such as mental health clinics, where more specialized individual treatment is available.[16]

There are two essential aspects of the dynamics of groups: the interpersonal relationships, making up the group process, and the task functions that constitute the group product. Interactions of members make groups go round, "sometimes fair and sometimes sour." Three basic processes are at work in interpersonal interactions: (1) inclusion: who is in and who is out; (2) dominance: who is on top, who is at the bottom, and who is in-between; and (3) closeness: who turns toward whom, who turns away, or who turns against others. These are oversimplified versions of many theoretical concepts developed in small-group research. In addition to developing interpersonal relationships the work of the group has to get done. The *work* (task) may be talking, feeling, learning, doing, playing. Through both, the interpersonal relationships and the tasks that people work on, a sense of "self," a self-image, emerges because people incorporate the reflection of others into their own self-perception.[17]

Access and Assistance Services

Transportation. As stated, the elderly face many transportation problems because they lack financial resources and often do not have access to facilities. Communities are beginning to provide greater mobility to older persons through reduction of fares for senior citizens. The lack of easily accessible routes and fears for personal safety, especially in urban areas, have become major problems. Many communities have introduced senior shuttle buses to make it easier for older persons to travel from one area of the community to another. This is usually arranged by an agency in cooperation with a municipality. Cab services have also been contracted to facilitate access to agencies, hospitals, clinics, or recreation and religious programs.

Information and Referral Services. Information and referral services are designed to provide information to individuals and agencies and to speed access to services for persons who are incapacitated, handicapped, or ill. The services also assemble important data used to evaluate community needs or gaps in services and resources. More than two hundred special information and referral service agencies have been organized in large communities by welfare councils, their affiliated social agencies, and by councils on aging. The nationwide public welfare program, however, does not provide a service that deals with the complicated problems people may have in using community service. Public welfare departments can provide information to public-assistance clients if staff is available. Many older people find it difficult to utilize information and referral services, and the majority of the aged are not even aware of their existence. In some instances, (for example, in Worcester, Massachusetts) it has been found that some older people utilizing information and referral services were really in need of highly skilled treatment services that were not immediately available.

Consumer Information. Most older persons have less disposable income than younger persons; yet they are often the targets of advertisements and promotions that are fraudulent. A number of federal agencies are working together to pool information for older people. Relatively little of this has filtered down to the community level as yet. The right to safety, the right to be informed, the right to be heard, and the right to choose are basic consumer rights. These are particularly important to older persons who tend to be more vulnerable to, and less able to afford the financial hardship of, fraud and deception in the marketplace. Vigorous action to protect the elderly against fraud and deceit is needed but especially with respect to those goods and services of which the elderly are disproportionate consumers.

In designing and implementing programs to protect the four basic consumer rights, the elderly, one of the fastest growing consumer subgroups, deserve special consideration. In particular, the development of effective consumer education and information programs is vital if older persons are to know about and understand the protections, rights, and remedies available to them.

Home-Repair Services. For older persons living alone, or for older couples, one of the critical issues (both in decaying urban centers and in rural areas) is the upkeep of property. Because of a lack of ability or of resources older persons may be living under hazardous conditions. Increasing attention is being given to the development of home-repair services whereby older persons, often retirees, are employed part-time to provide minor repair and household-maintenance services on the open market. This service includes a broad range of maintenance activities, such as plumbing, electrical, heating, painting, and roofing.

Respite Services. An emerging service focuses on relieving primary care takers, often children, spouses, or other relatives, and friends, of their day-to-day responsibilities for an older adult. Respite service is short-term care for the elderly during periods when no one is available to attend their needs. This program initiated in Sweden and is now offered at a number of geriatric-care centers in communities across the country.

Legal Services. One of the fastest developing services for older persons is assistance with special legal needs. Some legal issues are in the areas of consumer rights and protection, and others are in the more specialized areas of guardianship, conservatorship, and protective services. The civil rights of older persons and the need for legal advocacy is only now beginning to develop and become recognized as a component of social services.

Protective Services. These offer assistance to older people who may need help in managing their money or have fears of daily living but do not yet need the elaborate legal protection of a court-appointed guardian or conservatorships. They are defined as a "constellation of social services that assist older people who manifest a degree of incapacity or limited mental, emotional or physical function which may result in harm or hazard to themselves or others by helping individuals to continue to remain at a level of competence and function that will enable them to manage their own affairs."[18]

Protection for the elderly is to be sought and provided for in four areas: (1) protection of the life and property of the marginally functioning, noninstitutionalized elderly; (2) protection of civil liberties of these same elderly; (3) protection for professional persons working in this field, to free them from burdens of anxiety about their authority and its limits; (4) protection for the community from dangers posed by the incapacitated person. The National Council on Aging originally, and the National Council of Senior Centers later, spearheaded these services through their Legal Research and Services for the Elderly Project in 1968, which has resulted in legal-aid services to older people in the community. In 1973, Congress added these to those available under the Older Americans Act, and in 1975 legal services was established as one of the four national-priority services.[19]

Some definitions are useful here: *civil commitment* is a process whereby a person is committed (either voluntarily or involuntarily) to a state mental hospital. *Guardianship* is a legal device whereby decision-making power over one person's property or personal affairs is given to another on a legal finding of "incompetency" of the first person. *Protective services and emergency intervention*: some state laws have recognized the need to authorize "limited legal intervention" in certain situations not necessitating commitment or guardianship. These laws are designed to assist social workers, police, and the community in dealing with situations more temporary and less severe than those requiring guardianship or commitment. Other legal devices that provide for problems of property management include the power of attorney, trust, joint tenancy, and substitute payeeship.[20]

Peer-Group Outreach. Peer-group outreach is a social-support service that uses volunteers for case finding, then links individuals with existing health and social service resources. The elderly themselves provide volunteer services making use of their own skills and capacities. They serve as "buddies," social-group leaders, and friendly visitors. Working on a case finding offers older persons a potential for regaining lost confidence.

Volunteers at any age are a major resource for outreach as well as for direct services, especially for people who otherwise might be in institutions. This is particularly true of the Friendly Visitors Program, one of the oldest of the services. Volunteers, or paid professionals, visit to offer the older person companionship, a chat, social and recreational opportunities. In some instances, the roles of friendly visitor, home maker, and chore service are embodied in one person.

Health, social-supportive, and access services have been designed to assist older persons to stay in familiar surroundings. No one service can accomplish this alone, but a combination of the services can make this more of a reality. This enumeration of services is by no means exhaustive. New initiatives emerge continuously in many parts of the country as numerous governmental brochures, announcements, and privately sponsored publications attest.

Closed Care

Social services are offered in a number of long-term-care facilities, day-care centers, nursing homes, and rehabilitation centers as part of medically and/or custodially oriented institutions. Generally, social services constitute a small part of these institutions, although the Hebrew Rehabilitation Center of the Aged in Boston or the Hebrew Home for the Aged and Infirm in New York, among many others, have sizable social service departments and offer their residents many different types of services, notably recreation, group counseling, and case management. They also provide an important service link to family members of the older residents.

Many of the services listed before are also provided in institutions, although there are enormous gaps and deficiencies.

Delivery of Social Services

The overall objective of delivering social services is often phrased in terms of "maintaining an older person's independence." This is misleading. It is not a matter of maintaining independence, but rather of shifting some dependencies (notably social) from family to social service agencies. Community-based social services are attempts to allow elderly persons to remain in their community and out of institutions such as nursing homes or state hospitals. Independence for the elderly, then, is often synonymous with being not institutionalized. Interests other than those of the elderly are also served through a community social service approach. The elderly are spared the problems of living in impersonal institutions. The taxpayers are spared the cost of running such institutions.

As an example, let us look at a common problem among the elderly, nutrition, and one response of the society to this problem—congregate-dining facilities and meals on wheels. Many older persons live alone and on fixed income. Cooking an entire meal for one often hardly seems worth the cost and effort. As a result, many elderly persons suffer nutritional deficiencies. Over a period of time nutritional deficiencies lead to more serious health problems. Offering a community-based meals program therefore not only makes sense from the point of view of the elderly person but also for those who would have to pay for the far more expensive health care that would otherwise be required.

The same logic applies to the provision of home maker and chore services. Elderly persons may sometimes be unable to do their own housecleaning or laundry, but it would be neither in their own nor in the rest of society's interests to institutionalize them for these reasons. A homemaker can come into the older person's house several times each week at a fraction of the cost of institutional care. Home-health-aide programs provide a parallel service for the care of the older person's body. Baths, backrubs, and simple treatments such as changing dressings on wounds provide care that might otherwise be neglected. Some communities also have home-repair services that take care of such problems as broken windows, loose doorsteps, and leaky faucets or roofs.

Day-care programs for the elderly are perhaps the most intensive services available outside of institutionalizations. Day-care provides up to eight hours per day, five days a week of psychiatric, social, and rehabilitation services. Transportation to and from the day-care program is often provided, and participants eat one or more meals at the day-care center. These people may not be institutionalized on a twenty-four-hour basis, but they are certainly not independent in the usual sense of the word.

For many elderly persons their lack of a support system is better described as isolation than as dependency. Social isolation, that is, the lack of a support system, is a common problem among older people. Although it certainly is not true that all older persons are isolated, too often friends and family have frequently moved or died and the older person is left without needed human contact. Isolation, like nutritional deficits, leads to other problems. Therefore a number of social service programs have, either as a primary or secondary goal, the reduction of social isolation. Transportation services in vehicles designed to carry older passengers provide an important bridge between the elderly and the rest of the community. Activities programs are specifically designed to bring older people together for friendly social interaction. There are also a number of information and referral services that attempt to locate the isolated elderly and to put them in touch with other needed services. Even meal programs are designed to encourage social interaction. Ninety percent of the meals served through a nutrition program must be served in a congregate-dining facility; only 10 percent of the meals can be delivered to the older person's home, and then only if the person is physically unable to come to the dining facility.

Programs designed to reduce social isolation, as well as other services to the elderly, need to be flexibly planned and delivered to be sensitive to the differential needs of individual people. Too often old people are thought of as "all the same." There is no reason to believe that cultural or ethnic or religious differences, for example, disappear when people turn 65. The meals program that serves pork chops to its Jewish diners or the activities program that plans an evening of bingo for those whose religion prohibits gambling is likely to offend people and discourage further program participation.

There are also important age differences among those who are considered old, and social service programs need to reflect an awareness of these differences. The difference between the needs of a 60-year-old person and an 80-year-old person is often as great as the needs differences of 20 versus 40 year old persons.

Socialization is a process through which people learn to take part in new social situations. Through the process of socialization, children learn the "do's" and "don't's" of their culture. "Do" obey your parents and "don't" break rules. "Do" work hard and "don't" be a loafer. Above all "do" something "don't" just sit there. As every child who has attempted to idly sit in a classroom knows, "doing" something is itself an important American value. Americans ridicule members of this and other cultures who do not share the dominant preoccupation with activity. Consider the typical American jokes about meditating or Mexican siestas. Both are ridiculed as pursuits of the lazy. There is no value in America in just "being," one must "do."[21] Yet for older persons things are completely reversed. Their social situation requires that they stop "doing" and content themselves with just existing. Small wonder that special programs are required to socialize older people for the inactivity expected of them in later life.

Socialization for independence and individual hard work also creates other problems for older Americans and those who attempt to help older persons. Many elderly people's pride is often so tied up with self-reliance that even when they are very much in need, many will refuse help, and available programs or services are simply not acceptable. Refusing services is not an uncommon occurrence among the elderly. Part of the reason for this is the emphasis on independence and self-reliance in this society.

There are significant barriers to the delivery of services that are related not to their acceptability but rather to the practice of ageism. Robert Butler sums it up in the following way:

All types of services organization, whether voluntary non-profit, governmental or commercial, have tended to neglect older people. Only one-third of all the voluntary non-profit agencies of the United States can even claim to have special programs for the aged. Older people have had little influence upon these agencies, whose "accountability" derives largely from self-selected boards of trustees, even though 80 percent of their budgets comes from public donations. A substantial percentage of the dollars contributed to voluntary organizations through community drives (such as United Givers Funds and Community Chests) goes into overhead and administration, and what is left over is allocated to the actual provision of services. A miniscule amount of this goes to the elderly . . . non-profit foundations also illustrate institutionalized "ageism" by seldom providing money for use on behalf of the elderly. In rare instances where funding has occurred, little of lasting value has resulted. . . . Commercial providers such as businesses that offer nursing, companion and housekeeping service are no better, and in some ways far worse, than voluntary agencies. Since these are profit-making operations, accountability in the commercial service industries is largely confined to one or several owners or to a large number of stockholders. If the accountant says the company is in the red, the quality and quantity of services will diminish. As in any other business, decisions are made primarily on the basis of the debit sheet and the need for specific kinds of quality services becomes subordinated to profit and loss.[22]

Services follow a predictable course. They are delivered the most to those who need them the least. Eligibility requirements stigmatize recipients and anger nonrecipients; yet if there are no eligibility limits the middle- and higher-income population tends to make the greatest use of services while the disadvantaged and undereducated poor get overlooked. When programs focus on the poor, one runs into a troublesome facet of the Protestant Ethic that demands that "the deserving poor" be separated from the "undeserving." More than half of the poor are either over 65 or under 16, yet the image of the welfare recipient as a shiftless and lazy able-bodied adult persists as a major hinderance to provision of services.

Age discrimination in various federally funded programs is widespread. The U.S. Civil Rights Commission's 1977 Age Discrimination Study found age-based discrimination in numerous programs of importance to the elderly. The most pernicious of the causes of this pattern of discrimination is the tendency of program managers to target service delivery on younger persons on the theory that older people do not represent a wise investment of scarce resources.

Several 1978 amendments have strengthened the Age Discrimination Act. An important one provides victims of discriminatory practices with access of federal courts. Unfortunately, the ADA still permits federally supported programs to use discriminatory age criteria if it promotes a business or program objective. This is a loophole that will perpetuate discriminatory practices. Given the pervasiveness of age discrimination and in order to realize the Age Discrimination Act's stated goal, the ADA should be amended to limit the exclusionary use of age criteria to programs where federal statutes explicitly authorize the use of such criteria.[23]

Tobin and Lieberman offer alternative ways of structuring the delivery of services based on a continuum and a locus, either home-delivered or congregate-delivered (see table 7-1).[24] Tobin and Lieberman have also outlined a series of service-delivery issues, some of which are addressed in the following section.[25]

Major Issues in Social Service Delivery and Proposals

Even if a continuum of service delivery was commonly agreed upon and implemented, there are a number of structural issues that have to be resolved.

Table 7-1
Alternative Ways of Structuring the Delivery of Services

Continuum of Service	Home-Delivered (Client lives at home)	Congregate-Delivered	
		Congregate-Organized (Client lives at home)	Congregate Residence (Client lives at service site)
Services for the comparatively well elderly	Outreach Information and referral Telephone reassurance Friendly visiting Work at home Senior wheels to: shopping, doctor, dentist, and social functions	Adult education Recreational senior center Nutrition sites (wheels to meals) Sheltered workshops	Senior housing (includes retirement hotels) Senior housing with recreation and social services
Services that provide alternatives for preventing premature institutionalization	Escort service Homemaker service (housekeeping, handyman, etc.) Meals on wheels Home-health care (visiting nurse, rehabilitation, speech therapy, dentist, and doctor) Foster-home care (complete social and health care for bed-ridden person in a home)	Multipurpose senior center (all the above, plus outreach, health, and social follow-up)	Sheltered care Halfway houses
Services for those whose needs may demand institutional care or its equivalent		Outpatient day or hospital care	Mental hospital Institutional care (nursing homes and homes for the aged) intermediate-nursing care; skilled-nursing care; short-term crisis care; and vacation plan Terminal care

Source: Sheldon S. Robin and Morton A. Lieberman, *Last Home for the Aged* (San Francisco, Calif.: Jossey-Bass, Inc., 1976). Reprinted with permission of Jossey-Bass, Inc., Publishers.

What degree of comprehensiveness can a system achieve is one major question. Comprehensive services can be advocated because they address the total range of need, whereas fewer services provide intensive use of limited resources, are easier to implement, and promote development of expertise related to specific needs or problems. A compromise model would be a comprehensive system (1) capable of responding to a full range of service, (2) built around a case-management approach, (3) with agencies maintaining their own limited and expert focus.

A second structural issue relates to centralization versus decentralization of services and locus of authority. A compromise model is decentralized service delivery with centralized planning and resource allocation that makes services more accessible, capitalizes on the informal helping network, and also increases local autonomy.

The third question relates to coordination versus autonomy: how can the functional relationship maximize the range of client services? Coordinated services strengthen agencies' capacities to deliver service effectively and promote specialization and refinement. On the other hand, coordination among agencies may be difficult to arrange. Autonomy allows for organizational structures that are simpler and easier to control. A middle course may be to link autonomous units closely enough to assure that clients move smoothly through the system.

In addition to structural issues there are three major client considerations. First the well-known age-integrated versus age-segregated argument rears its head. Should the elderly be served separately from other age groups? It can be argued that the elderly have special problems requiring the bringing together of specialists, that the elderly tend to lose out when mixed with other age groups, and that they are strengthened by peer interaction. Arguing against age segregation are lower costs of delivering services when persons of various ages can share them, and avoidance of age segregation. A possible solution might be to offer age-segregated services, with linkages to age-free services. It is possible that concentration of older persons in their own communities is by far the most economical way to serve them, allowing for special transportation, ready availability of day hospitals, and health centers staffed with specialists in medical gerontology, specialists in rehabilitation, and nursing.

Greater economy might possibly be achieved through integration of older persons into other social service networks through exchange of child care and elderly care in intergenerational families, or—for fees—among families not related. Subcommunities for older persons within larger integrated communities, which might allow them to have the benefits of both approaches (as long as the distances are not too large) might also be explored.[26]

The existence of a sizable, vulnerable, frail elderly population points to another major issue: to what extent shall resources (and services) be allocated to those who are more at-risk rather than to those who are less impaired?

The Federal Council's 1978 Report "Public Policy and the Frail Elderly," addressed this issue and made the following proposal for services to the frail elderly[27]:

> The Council's recommendation for systematizing aid to persons who need direct personal assistance from society on a continuing basis is for a free-standing case assessment and case management service as an entitlement to the frail elderly upon reaching a certain age, on a national and voluntary basis. Frail persons below the age set could be qualified by some functional eligibility determination. This essentially social model should be complementary and of equal stature to services designed to meet the long-term health care needs of this population.
>
> This "floor" of social services would provide a skilled practitioner to develop a plan of care in conjunction with the older person and his or her family and/or friends. A priority in the assessment and plan process would be identification of a "significant other person" (or persons) available to the frail older person to assist in coping with daily needs. The practitioner should see to the provision of such a "significant other" if none were already available. Case management would be an on-going service—its intensity dependent upon the needs and wishes of the older person and his or her family and/or friends.[28]

This proposal is based on the following eight principles:

1. There are many persons within the aging populations who, because of an accumulation of various continuing problems, require the assistance of a significant person from time to time to aid in coping with certain daily life activities.

2. Where there is limited or no continuing availability of a significant person, certain aids for life management should be assured by government if agreed to by the frail person.

3. The Federal Council on the Aging proposes that this assistance be available on a universal basis, as an entitlement, and be primarily of a social-support nature consisting of the following services: case assessment, plan of care, and case management.

4. The core services should be available on the basis of presumptive eligibility, determined on the basis of attaining a certain age; 75, for instance. Persons below that defined age with need for these services should have access through some form of functional assessment.

5. The core services should be administered by a single state agency with federal and state matching funding and flexible delivery at the community level.

6. When a significant person is not available or has not been identified through case assessment, priority in developing the plan of care should be given to the provision of such a person.

7. Any other services identified as being needed or desired are to be obtained from informal or formal services and all benefits made available to older persons.

8. A mechanism should be developed for providing data about the unmet needs of the frail elderly to community planning agencies and leadership and advocacy groups.[29]

The report goes on to advocate improvements in income, health, housing and social service for all the elderly. It states that:

> The Council believes there should be no let up in efforts to assure that all older Americans have sufficient material resources and sound health aid in order that they may continue "the pursuit of happiness" throughout the longest of lives and adopted a resolution requesting the Chairman to propose a coordinated effort at the highest level of government for developing long-term care policy in the United States.[30]

In deciding on service arrangements, one has to balance the virtues of home-delivered approaches (serving people in familiar, nonthreatening environments and avoiding stressful relocation), against those of congregate approaches (the positive effects of peer socialization, promotion of a positive aging image, and lower costs). A mix of graduated services—with mechanisms for service integration (for example, multipurpose centers and case managers) that can provide alternatives to institutional care—is often the best compromise.

In addition to ageist attitudes there are also sexist and racist attitudes that have created further barriers to the provision and delivery of social services, usually referred to as constituting double and triple jeopardy.

Older Women

Older women are a majority of the population age 65 and over. By the year 2000 they will represent 60 percent of that population. Moreover, as the 75 + and 85 + segments grow, the proportion of women in those segments will grow even faster because of longer life expectancy. Policy must begin to reflect the impact of this aspect of the demographic trend in the design of programs.

Many older women live alone or with nonrelatives. A large proportion are in poverty. The income they do have tends to come from public programs like social security or SSI. Only 8 percent are in the labor force. To help relieve their adverse income situation, older women need opportunities for income supplementation. The creation of such opportunities requires that stereotypes of older women that have been barriers to their employment be changed, nontraditional work schedules like "flexi-time" be implemented, and economic disincentives, such as social security's earnings limitation, be removed. Finally the public and private retirement systems as well as social security must be reshaped so that women contribute as equals and derive benefits equal to those of men.

In addition to the problem of inadequate income, older women must deal with a host of social and psychological problems. Widowhood, late-life divorce, or separation leave many groping for an independence they are ill-equipped to pursue. Programs designed to assist older women who find themselves in such situations must be developed and funded. Increased enforcement of statutes such as the Equal Credit Opportunity Act will help by providing protection against unwarranted discrimination. But no matter what specific actions are pursued, the cumulative impact must be a reversal of society's negative image of women in general.[31]

Racism and Older People

The elderly are a multiracial and multicultural group. Many are immigrants from other countries. At least 1.6 million are persons of minority group background—blacks, Indians, Cubans, Mexican Americans, Puerto Ricans, Asian Americans. A nation as diverse as the United States needs transcultural studies of the elderly within its own borders; different cultural and racial groups have different conceptions of the life cycle; each has been treated somewhat differently by the majority white culture.

There are two major and distinctly separate issues regarding minority-group elderly. First are the unique cultural elements found in each minority group, which have bearing on the lives of its elderly members; second are the effects imposed on the elderly as a result of living in a majority white culture.

The prevailing racist attitudes exemplified in social institutions have created additional barriers in reaching nonwhite older persons through existing social service programs. Our discriminating practices, despite avowed statements to the contrary, leave more nonwhite elderly unserved than white elderly. Only strict adherence to affirmative action programs will make dents for the present aging cohorts, and only massive efforts by social activists, legislators, and planners jointly will bring about nondiscriminatory social policies for future cohorts.[32]

The double jeopardy effect on nonwhite aged has entered the consciousness of policy designers, planners, and practitioners. The backgrounds of older people based on their racial and ethnic heritage in a pluralistic society must allow for different responses by public social policies. This is particularly true for people from different immigration groups, such as those who arrived recently as older people from European or Asian countries as well as those who have grown older here as members of first immigrant generations that arrived in the late nineteenth and early twentieth centuries. To what extent do ethnic heritages, embodied in cultural values, ideologies, and traditions reflect and affect the view of the aged themselves, and to what extent are these aspects truly considered in the design and implementation of public policies?[33]

Besides client and structural issues there are also *strategic* issues in the delivery of services. First there is the issue of public versus private auspices. The many pros and cons lead to suggesting a system where planning is in accord with local political realities and where service delivery draws on the specialized abilities of different providers to fill service and organizational goals.

A second question relates to direct provisions versus purchase of service from other agencies. A combination of purchase and provision arrangements that promote effectiveness through competition while allowing for semiautonomous functioning, that assure the client of service while enhancing personal choice, and that also provide for the minority elderly's special needs may be most sensible but also most difficult to achieve.

Last but not least is the question of the nature of service providers themselves. Professional and paraprofessionals make up the majority of the social service work force. Social workers, home-health-care workers, practical nurses, recreation specialists, and adult educators, volunteers of all ages, constitute this service network. In addition, there are the relatives, friends, neighbors, and peers who constitute the informal (natural) network of helpers. Even with formal, organized social help and change efforts—and, sometimes, despite these efforts—informal systems of help in addition to family efforts have continued to flourish in almost all communities. Recent studies have concluded that an informal social support system, a natural helping network, exists for the elderly.[34] This network helps to sustain elderly people both emotionally and physically and acts as a supplement to the formal system, which often does not adequately meet their needs. It was found that informal service providers, relatives, friends, and neighbors are frequently the primary support system of elderly people. They provide the linkage between the older person and needed social and health services.

However, the natural neighbor-helper may see the representative of the formal helping agency as an intruder. The professional may have difficulty in moving away from traditional service-delivery techniques to work in a peer relationship in an unstructured situation. Therefore, a high level of professional training and discipline is necessary to strengthen the natural system without disrupting its delicate balance.

Arguing for the use of professionals is the higher skill level and the capacity to function independently; arguing for nonprofessionals and for volunteers is the promotion of effective linkages to community and natural helping systems, and the savings in cost—although training and supervision are not without costs. It may be preferable to have a mix of staff that includes a sufficient number of professionals to accomplish agency goals as well as volunteers and natural helpers who provide for cost-saving services and promote important community linkages.

Despite such preferred arrangements older persons are faced with an enlarged service bureaucracy and their lives are affected by this phenomenon. Service bureaucracies are organized along hierarchical lines with formal roles, that is, director, supervisor, staff worker. Each person has a specific task to perform and is subordinate to those higher up in the hierarchy. Bureaucracies are also characterized by formal rules and regulations for their operation. Human service workers who come in face-to-face contact with elderly clients are expected to adhere to these rules in providing services to their clients. Older persons whose lives come into frequent contact with service bureaucracies thus spend a good deal of their time dealing with red tape. The elderly client, whose income is just over the cut-off limit, or the one who wants to discuss his problems now but has to wait until the next scheduled counseling session, experiences a frustration known only to those who must live according to the rules and timetables of service bureaucracies. One aged woman, living in a New York City "welfare" hotel, puts it this way:

> This is my social life, . . . I run around the city and stand in line . . . I stand in line for medicine, for food, for glasses, for the cards to get pills, for the pills; I stand in line to see people who never see who I am; at the hotels, sometimes I even have to stand in line to go to the john. When I die there'll probably be a line to get through the gate, and when I get up to the front of the line, somebody will push it closed and say, "Sorry, come back after lunch." These agencies I figure they have to make it as hard for you to get help as they can, so only really strong people or really stubborn people like me can survive. All the rest die; standing in line.[35]

Bureaucracies develop a life of their own, continuing to operate even if they serve poorly those for whom they were created. It is important to realize that there are often conflicts between maintaining an agency and providing the best possible services. We have all heard stories of the hospital patient who died while waiting for the insurance forms to be completed![36]

For social service agencies to obtain or maintain government funding they must often demonstrate high "success rates" based on quantified data. Let us assume that one of the criteria for the continued funding of a day-care center for the aged is that 80 percent of those patients taken into the program will remain living in the community and will be kept out of twenty-four-hour institutions. To meet this 80 percent success rate, the director issues a policy statement that elderly applicants whose problems are very serious and are at risk of entering a twenty-four-hour institution should not be allowed to enter the day-care program. Thus to maintain itself, the organization avoids difficult cases. We are thus confronted with the paradox that those elderly who are most in need of a day-care program to head off possible institutionalization are least likely to receive that service.

Perhaps, though, the greatest danger of the bureaucratization is the threat posed to the freedom of older people. There are times when bureaucracies must be opposed, and this opposition can come only from autonomous people who are strong enough to stand up to the "powers that be." Who shall decide what, if any service is best? Professionals, because of their training and skill, claim legitimate authority in these decisions. Family members, because of their long involvement with and love for an older relative, often believe that they are in a position to know what is best for their mothers, fathers, aunts, and uncles. Elderly clients themselves may believe that only they can determine what course of action is in their best interests. If all the parties agree, for example, that daily participation in a congregate-dining program and weekly participation in an activities program is ideal, then there is no issue. However, what if only the social worker believes that this is a desirable plan? The elderly client may wish to have meals delivered home and have nothing to do with congregate-dining or activities programs. The family may be concerned about their older relative living alone and feel that supervised housing is required. Who has legitimate authority in this case? Suffice to say that the issues involved in answering this question are larger than the individuals caught up in these situations. Individual freedom and self-determination are basic values in this society. Placing control of someone's life in the hands of either a professional or a relative can have important social as well as personal consequences. For instance, a study documents these problems: An elderly lady was convinced by a psychiatric resident to come to Central State Hospital for an "evaluation," and upon arrival was committed. A confused elderly apartment dweller was admitted to the medical hospital for observation after a fall and later discharged to a nursing home without ever being told she was not going home.[37]

Individual freedom becomes a particularly critical issue in protective services for the elderly. Many elderly persons may need help in managing a budget or other aspects of their daily lives. Their limitations are not serious enough to warrant the appointment of a legal guardian, but mental or physical handicaps threaten their independent functioning. A social worker takes responsibility for making many of the decisions about money allocation, housing, arrangements, social activities, or other decisions usually considered the domain of the individual. Older persons who accept these services have in a sense publically admitted that they are incapable of managing important areas of their lives. How then, if there is a disagreement between the social worker and the client, can the client maintain autonomy in the disputed area? Does the individual have to relinquish freedom in return for the care and protection provided?

A similar development might be expected as service bureaucracies expand into more aspects of the older person's life. The elderly client who is dependent on a social agency for transportation, meals, and health care might have difficulty in opposing a social worker's decision to change the client's housing arrangements. Both social workers and elderly clients must be cautious and circumspect in dealing with the shift in decision-making power precipitated by the expansion of service bureaucracies for the aged. The importance of older persons participating in the planning process, as well as in the decisions affecting how services shall be organized and delivered to meet their needs cannot be overemphasized. Advocacy efforts and involvement by older people themselves in planning and implementation of programs on an organized and ad-hoc basis is a direct outgrowth of this concern and can be a major factor in redressing the balance toward more equitable power on the part of the aged.

Models for Social Service Planning

A number of models for service planning have been suggested that warrant discussion and monitored evaluation. Stanley Brody in promoting the health and social service system model argues that medical care is but one important part of the continuum of health care and that health and social services are equally important and "not ancillary" to any other service. He suggests that the parallel functions be met by the health and social service system in both the community and the inpatient, acute hospital. These include: personal services; supportive or extended medical services; maintenance services; counseling—including listening skills and the mobilization and utilization of resources; and linkage services (information, referral, and education).[38]

Elaine Brody emphasizes the developmental model, which stresses that there are tasks to be mastered in the later stages of life as in the earlier phases. This view recognizes the range of differences within the aging stage of life and the "unique potentials" of psychological well-being for older persons. She further suggests that the developmental concept brings into focus the need to critically examine the usefulness and appropriateness of knowledge and techniques borrowed from work with the young.[39]

Robert Morris proposes a service-delivery approach to respond to the needs of the long-term sick, handicapped, and disabled, with the elderly representing the largest majority of this population. Morris points out that medical and social agencies seldom consider the slow-moving long-term case as their primary responsibility; they are to be "referred" to some "other agency" for social, economic, and psychological conditions. Because no other agency can or is willing to take such sustained responsibility, such individuals end up in inappropriate institutions, such as nursing homes, which cannot meet their needs. His proposal is for a personal care service system model to maximize residential choice for the elderly and disabled. Such a service system, he argues, would decrease inappropriate institutionalization and optimize the functional capacities of such individuals in the housing and neighborhoods of their preference.[40]

Sheldon Tobin believes that there are likely to emerge community based social and health service systems that will provide for continuing supportive care as the individual's needs change. Therefore, he suggests that neighborhood-based centers, placing a priority on services to the aging, will emerge out of higher expectations and demands of older persons and the increased sensitivity to their needs by service providers. This will be part of the local primary-care system backed up by small local institutions developed by those responsible for the local neighborhood-care systems. This would allow for a more decentralized approach, keeping the majority of older persons in their familiar habitat and environment.[41]

Lowy suggests a supermarket-of-services model for delivery on the local level. State units on aging would have responsibility to provide a broad range of services and arrangements to meet the needs of the elderly, including meals, recreation, information and outreach, transportation facilities, boarding homes, visiting and social work services, and home facilities on a local level.[42] In addition, to bring about the closest integration between health and social services, older people are to be provided with health care services, home-health aids, meals, sheltered care, mental health screening, and treatment on a mobile basis, if needed. Each state agency on aging would be vested with authority to develop one-stop local service centers with maximum input by consumers of services to develop, design, administer, and deliver such services. Each local center—geographically accessible to the older population—would be accountable to a board and this board, in turn, to the state agency on aging.

The AOA would provide guidelines and funding to the state unit on aging, responsible directly to the governor's office. AOA, in fact, would be the national service agency for all programs for older persons and have statutory responsibility for connecting all federal departments on behalf of the aged.

The local agencies would indeed by expected to relate the informal network to the formal network and to bring to bear a wholistic approach to service delivery in the community to be integrated by the agency and not by the clients.[43]

Kamerman, in a cross-national study of eight countries concludes that the major users of services other than the socialization and recreational services are those aged 75 and older; the most heavily used services, where available, involve a mix of health and social services. In those countries where they are available, a cluster of home-based personal-care services (or social care) have been identified as critical for helping the aged remain in their own homes or in congregate housing. Regardless of whether these services are provided in ordinary or specially designed housing, the important common theme is the element of practical care and help.

Although the importance of this category of services is obvious in every country, a delivery structure organized around providing these services has not yet emerged. Some are provided under medical auspices; others under social welfare auspices; but rarely are they available in one place, under an integrated delivery structure. Except in the United Kingdom, there is no realization that these personal-care services should be the focal point of any community service system for the aged and that stressing this personal-care function could improve service delivery generally, making it far more responsive to the needs of the aged. Personal-care services are identifiable, concrete aids and represent the key to achieving a major objective: supporting the aged in comfort and dignity, be it in their own home, another's home, or a special facility.[44]

Social services are an integral component of any supportive service system. Both individual and group services are to be provided for older persons. Social workers should have an active leadership role in the planning and provision of social services. Programs should utilize the natural helping network and integrate it with the formal, bureaucratic structures that need to be responsive to individual human needs and concerns. The social service system must provide for consumer choice and participation in the use of services, for the protection of individuality, and for participation in policy making. Based on the concept of self-determination, consumers should have the right to receive or refuse services without penalty, thus acknowledging individual responsibility and judgment. Confidentiality of information and other consumer rights must be safeguarded. Effective participation must be guaranteed by the provision of training, education, and opportunities for decision making by the elderly.

There also must be mechanisms to provide maximum accountability. Funding sources, policy-making bodies, administrators, service personnel, and consumers should obtain regular and precise information as to the operations, trends, problems, and results of service delivery. Built-in provisions for rapid retrieval of data to monitor the quality and quantity of services must be provided. Financing must be secured through federal funds. Various financing methods are now in effect under various titles, such as Title XX (SSA) and Title III (OAA)—governmental- and voluntarily financed free services where there is a large or special stake in the utilization; insurance financed, prepaid services involving time-limited defined-risk situations; and purchase of governmental, voluntary, and entrepreneur services involving individual responsibility, and other variations. Under present political conditions, a variable financing program will be a transition necessity. However, in the not-too-distant future, a universal system with no financial barriers to social services—not only for the poor and needy—will have to be developed by the federal government, based on a progressive tax structure that will assure a more equitable fiscal distribution in accord with a philosophy of intergenerational solidarity.

Notes

1. Reports of White House conferences: U.S. Department of Health, Education and Welfare, *The Nation and Its Older People* (Washington, D.C., 1961); and U.S. Department of Health, Education and Welfare, *Toward a National Policy on Aging* (Washington, D.C., 1971); see also, Walter M. Beattie, Jr. "Aging and the Social Services" in R. Binstock and E. Shanas, eds., *Handbook of Aging and the Social Sciences* (New York: Van Nostrand, Reinhold, 1978), p. 619.

2. Abrahan H. Maslow, *Motivation and Personality* (New York: Harper and Row, 1954).

3. Robert H. Binstock and Martin A. Levin, "The Political Dilemma of Intervention Policies," in Robert H. Binstock and Ethel Shanas, eds., *Handbook of Aging and the Social Sciences* (New York: Van Nostrand, Reinhold, 1976).

4. Robert Hudson, "The Graying of the Federal Budget," *The Gerontologist* 18 (1978):428-439.

5. Talcott Parsons, "The Professions and Social Structure," *Social Forces* 17 (1939):457-467.

6. Margaret E. Kuhn, "Open Letter," *The Gerontologist* 18 (1978): 422-424.

7. Sheila Kamerman and Alfred Kahn, *Social Services in the United States* (Philadelphia: Temple University Press, 1976).

8. *Older Americans Act of 1965*, Title I. Administration on Aging, DHEW Publication, 1979.

9. Virginia Little, "Open Care for the Aging: Alternate Approaches," U.S. Department of Health, Education and Welfare, Administration on Aging (Washington, D.C., November-December 1979).

10. This material is based on categorizations developed by this author and described in his book *Social Work with the Aging* (New York: Harper & Row, 1979).

11. Elaine M. Brody, *A Social Work Guide for Long-Term Care Facilities* (Rockville, Md.: National Institute of Mental Health, 1974); Elaine M. Brody, "Aging," *Encyclopedia of Social Work* (Washington, D.C.: National Association of Social Workers, 1977); Elaine M. Brody,

"The Aging Family," *The Gerontologist* (6) (1966):4; and Margaret Blenkner, "Social Work and Family Relationships in Later Years with Some Thoughts on Filial Maturity," in Ethel Shanas and Gordan F. Streib, eds., *Social Structure and the Family: Generational Relations* (Englewood Cliffs, N.J.: Prentice-Hall, 1965).

12. L. Bellack and H. Barten, eds., *Progress in Community Mental Health* (N.Y.: Grune and Stratton, 1969).

13. National Council on the Aging, *Directory of Senior Centers and Clubs* (Washington, D.C., 1975).

14. Louis Lowy, "The Senior Center, a Community Facility," *Perspective*, vol. 3 no. 2, (March/April 1974), pp. 5-9.

15. *Lifeline, An Emergency Alarm System* (Report to the Health Care Finance Administration by Hebrew Rehabilitation Center for the Aged, Boston, 1980).

16. Lowy, *Social Work*, chap. 12, and Irene M. Burnside: *Working with the Elderly: Group Processes and Techniques* (Belmont, Calif., Duxbury Press, 1978).

17. Lowy, *Social Work*.

18. Gertrude H. Hall and Geneva Mathiasen, *Guide to Development of Protective Services for Older People* (Springfield, Ill.: Charles C. Thomas, Bannerstone House, 1973).

19. U.S., Congress, Senate, Special Committee on Aging, *Protective Services for the Elderly* (Paper prepared by John J. Regan and Georgia Springer, Washington, D.C., 1977).

20. *Law and Aging Manual* (Washington, D.C.: National Council of Senior Citizens, 1976), appendix.

21. Florence R. Kluckhohn, "Dominant and Variant Value Orientations," in Clyde Kluckhohn and Henry A. Murray, eds., *Personality in Nature, Society and Culture* (New York: Alfred Knopf, 1967), pp. 342-360.

22. Robert N. Butler, M.D., *Why Survive? Being Old in America* (New York: Harper and Row, 1975), pp. 159-162.

23. U.S. Civil Rights Commission, *Age Discrimination Study* (Washington, D.C., 1977).

24. Sheldon S. Tobin and Morton St. Lieberman, *Last Home for the Aged* (San Francisco: Jossey-Bass, 1976).

25. Ibid.

26. Amitai Etzioni, "Old People and Public Policy," *Social Policy* November/December 1976, p. 27.

27. U.S. Department of Health, Education and Welfare, Federal Council on Aging, *Public Policy and the Frail Elderly*, DHEW Publication (OHDS) 79-20959 (Washington, D.C., 1978).

28. Ibid., p. 8.

29. Ibid., p. 57.

30. Ibid., p. 58.

31. *No Longer Young: The Older Woman in America* (Work Group Reports from the 26th Conference on Aging, Institute of Gerontology, University of Michigan, Wayne State University, 1975); U.S., Congress, *Hearings before the Joint Economic Committee: Economic Problems of Women* (1971); U.S., Congress, House, House Select Committee on Aging, *Economic Problems of Aging Women—Hearings before the Subcommittee on Retirement, Income and Employment*, (1975); U.S., 9th Congress, 1st session House, Select Committee on Aging, Social Security Inequities against Women—*Hearings*, (1975).

32. Erdman Palmore and Kenneth Manton, "Ageism Compared to Racism and Sexism," in M. Seltzer, S. Corbett, and R. Atchley, eds., *Social Problems of the Aging* (Belmont, Calif.: Wadsworth Publishing, 1978); Human Resources Corporation, *Policy Issues Concerning the Minority Elderly*, contracted by the Federal Council on the Aging (Washington, D.C., 1978).

33. See "Aging and Ethnicity," in R.A. Kalish, ed., *The Later Years* (Monterey, Calif.: Brooks/Cole, 1977).

34. Marjorie H. Cantor, *The Elderly in the Inner City* (New York: New York City Office for the Aging, 1973); Anna H. Zimmer et al., *Incentives to Families Caring for Disabled Elderly: Research and Demonstration Project to Strengthen the Natural Supports System*, Community Service Society of New York (Presented at the 30th Annual Meeting of the Gerontological Society, San Francisco Hilton, November 1977).

35. Sharon R. Curtin. *Nobody Ever Died of Old Age* (Boston: Atlantic-Little, Brown Books, 1972).

36. Paul Paillat, "Bureaucratization of Old Age: Determinants of the Process, Possible Safeguards and Reorientation," Ethel Shanas and Marvin B. Sussman, eds., *Family Bureaucracy and the Elderly* (Durham, N.C.: Duke University Press, 1977).

37. Dwight Frankfather, *The Aged in the Community* (New York: Praeger, 1977).

38. Stanley J. Brody, "Comprehensive Health Care for the Elderly: An Analysis," *Gerontologist* 13 (1973):412-418.

39. Brody, "Aging," pp. 51-74.

40. Robert Morris and Delwin Anderson," Personal Care Services: An Identity for Social Work," *Social Service Review* (June 1975):157-174.

41. Sheldon S. Tobin, Stephen M. Davidson, and Ann Sack, *Effective Social Services for Older Americans* (Ann Arbor, Mich.: Institute of Gerontology, 1976).

42. Louis Lowy, "Models for Organization of Services to the Aging," *Aging and Human Development* 1 (1970):21-36.

43. Louis Lowy, "A Social Work Practice Perspective in Relation to Theoretical Models and Research in Gerontology," in Donald P. Kent, Robert Kastenbaum, and Sylvia Sherwood, eds., *Research Planning and Action for the Elderly* (New York: Behavioral Publications, 1972), pp. 538-544.

44. Sheila B. Kamerman, "Community Services for the Aged: The View from Eight Countries," *The Gerontologist* 16 (1976):529-537.

8 Organization and Participation of Older People

Older persons have become more politically as well as socially and physically active over the past two decades, and such political activism on the part of those over 65 has gained in legitimacy. Older persons perceive themselves as entitled to public participation as a group and as individuals, although they do not appear to have as yet developed a political self-image akin to politically organized ethnic groups. The question is to what extent public policy should encourage, discourage, or ignore these tendencies toward increased political activism on the part of older Americans.

At stake is a conception of what is to be deemed appropriate, democratically legitimate participation in public affairs. Thus, it has been stated about practically all active groups that they are not a "proper" base for public action. Behind this suggestion often is a textbook image of the democratic process: the government is run by elected representatives, and the legitimate way to influence them is by casting one's vote as a citizen and not as a member of any partisan group. Likewise, it is thought that voting preferences should be based on considerations of the nation's needs rather than on the needs or desire for special privileges of a particular subgroup.

Although it is quite true that, in part, the democratic process does work this way, it also proceeds by a large variety of groups each looking after its own set of concerns—not just "lobbies" or private-interest groups, such as farm, labor, or business groups, but groups promoting the civil rights of particular constituencies such as the NAACP, CORE, Italian American Association, American Jewish Congress, as well as groups representing the public interest such as the American Civil Liberties Union, Nader's Raiders, and so forth. Indeed, to the extent that the government does attend to the people's needs it works at least as much by responding to these groups, which among them encompass most Americans, as to general voters. It also follows that needs not so represented or weakly represented will tend to be underserved.

One might argue that the processes of government would be more rational and more ethical if there were no such groupings, but they exist in all societies, especially in democratic ones, and it is unrealistic to assume their demise, although one may seek to reduce their influence. Hence, for older persons, or any other group, to forgo collective action and participation in the competition for public awareness of and attention to their needs is basically to allow other groups to gain a larger share of the government attention and resources.

The question might be raised whether older persons have not already gained an excessive share of publicly allocated resources. This is perhaps the case where their "clout" is compared to some much weaker groups, such as the poor, the handicapped, and the mentally ill, but compared to the main power groups this seems hardly the case. Hence a greater political mobilization of older persons on behalf of the rights and needs of older persons both is quite legitimate and will serve to better balance the scale of allocative justice rather than bias it.

A phenomenon that emerged in the 1930s and continues today is the relatively widespread organization of older people on their own behalf. Grass-roots involvement and social-action commitment can bring about feelings of personal dignity, self-worth, and control over one's destiny and also create a deeper sense of accomplishment for a large group of older people. "Senior power" became a slogan in the late 1960s, and the Gray Panthers are, perhaps, one of the most significant illustrations of the translation of this slogan into practice. Their statement of purpose that they are a group of people, old and young, who are together because of deeply felt common concerns for human liberation and social change, expresses this particular philosophy well. The question of the politicization of older people and their assertion of their rights, particularly in view of a changing aging population based on differential acceptance of their status in society, may, in fact, move us further toward their assertion as a special-interest group. Several political scientists, notably Robert Binstock, are somewhat skeptical as to the viability, as well as to the ultimate gains, of such organizations.[1] Without minimizing the importance of organizations for those who are involved in it, he, and others, question whether, indeed, this is likely to transform American society and provide for the elderly a significant role.

Historical Perspective

The dramatic history of organizing for political ends dates back to the early 1930s. During this period the largest relief movement to that date had been initiated by Dr. Francis Townsend, although there were political stirrings long before that time.[2] Dr. Townsend had rallied thousands of people behind the demands of the elderly. He promoted the concept of a monthly pension of $250 for all citizens over 60 years of age to be paid on the conditions that they forgo gainful employment and that they spend every pension dollar within thirty days. The supporters of this scheme reasoned that the purchasing power created by giving the elderly a yearly income of $3000 would stimulate business and generate full employment, thus benefiting everyone. The movement attracted many people as the aged were hit hard by unemployment. By 1936, there were some 7,000 Townsend Clubs in the

United States, each with an average membership of 300. The Townsend group introduced its plan to Congress with 25 million signatures, but when the bill came to the Senate floor, over 200 congressmen did not show up. The liberals who did vote, voted the bill down without a roll call. But the Townsend people thought they did not fight in vain. They claimed that their advocacy had a lot to do with the eventual passage of the Social Security Act in 1935.

The National Association of Retired Federal Employees, founded in 1921, lobbied for the 1959 Federal Employees Health Benefit Law, but due to lack of numbers and growth of its organization, it related only marginally to broad legislative issues. Since then there have been only sporadic attempts by older people to organize until the 1961 White House Conference on Aging made the growing number of older people politically conscious and led to the creation of elderly organizations such as the American Association of Retired Persons and the National Retired Teachers Association, whose major focus is the improvement of the image and status of older people. Founded by Percy Andrews it is now the largest organization of its kind in the country. It has close ties with the insurance and business community. Its Legislative Council lobbies extensively in governmental offices and in the halls of Congress as well as in state legislatures for the adoption of legislation promoted by the leadership of the organization and ratified by its own constituent members. The National Council of Senior Citizens' (NCSC) initial goal was to generate pressure for the enactment of medicare. It built its constituency around vestiges of "the Senior Citizens for Kennedy" founded in 1960. It has significant ties to industrial unions.[3]

The National Caucus on the Black Aged was founded in 1970 to mitigate the dilution of the needs of black aged during the preparation for the 1971 White House Conference. Its principal objectives were to press for increased participation by blacks and for creating a special session at the conference to highlight the needs of aged blacks, because insufficient attention had been given to minorities in the formulation of issues and policy recommendations in the various pre-White House Conference meetings. In 1973 the National Caucus stimulated the creation of the National Center on the Black Aged, which not only fulfills advocacy functions but also provide programs of coordination, information, and consultation to meet the needs of black older people.

In June of 1970, Margaret (Maggie) Kuhn and five of her friends—all of whom were retiring from various national, religious, and social work agencies—came together to discuss the common problems that most retirees face: a degree of income loss, loss of contact with associates, and the loss of one of the most important identity-defining roles in this society, one's job. Despite the difficulties they faced, they had also acquired a new kind of freedom as retired people, which could be used to promote and support social goals for the elderly. They founded the Gray Panthers. In 1973, the Gray Panthers joined forces with the Retired Professional Action Group, which had been organized as one of Ralph Nader's public-citizen groups. This merger formalized the working relationships that the two groups had had since 1971 as organizations through which the talents, skills, and experiences of older people could be utilized. Both groups had attracted a nationwide constituency, older as well as younger people. The movement had become national in scope. There are now hundreds of local Gray Panther chapters in most states of the Union.[4]

In Massachusetts Frank Manning created the Massachusetts Legislative Council for Older Americans in 1963 to influence states and national political decisions on behalf of older persons.[5] In Minnesota and Ohio groups to draw attention to the plight of nursing-home residents were formed and became significant social-action advocates.

To what extent these organizations have significantly influenced national, state, and local policies is by no means established. Binstock points out that these aging organizations have sufficient power to maintain themselves and their interests, but the goals articulated and sought by these groups and the means at their disposal are not suitable and sufficient to redress fundamentally the economic, biomedical, and social problems of the severely disadvantaged aged, let alone change the general status of the aged. He notes that they have three forms of power: ready access to public officials; legitimacy to obtain public platforms; and electoral bluff, whereby public officials do not want to offend the aged and favor proposals providing some residual benefits.[6] Hudson in reviewing the current situation lists three factors that impede further progress: notably the growing cost of programs, the debate over distribution and needs, and competition for shrinking service funds.[7] In his estimation securing additional benefits will increasingly entail overcoming the presence of new resistance and the decline of the legitimacy and utility that have been the mainstays of political support. Monetary and opportunity costs have caught up with material benefits and perhaps even symbolic ones. Elected officials can no longer lend unquestioned support to aging initiatives, competing interests can no longer remain uninvolved, and budgetary officials on both the legislative and executive side may be decidedly hostile: ". . . Even if political pressure generated by the aging turns out to be relatively effective, a question remains as to what ends this pressure will be directed. It will be used if necessary—and probably successfully—to maintain policy gains already won. It is easier to defeat moves to rescind existing benefits than it is to gain enactment of new ones."[8]

As with all movements that become institutionalized, bureaucratization takes effect, and organizational imperatives, such as group maintenance, leadership struggles, and conflicts over goals, direction, and strategies become major agenda items. The activities of aging-based organizations in contemporary America are quite conservative; they are not radical or even left-liberal. However, the existence of a growing young-old population may throw new light on the political participation of the elderly. They presently constitute 15 percent of total population; women outnumber men; there are strong family ties with a large proportion having a living parent. Successive cohorts of the young-old are better educated and quite active as voters with more expectations of governmental responsibilities for the well-being of their generation. And those who are still in the labor force are likely to be affected by the conditions that obtain in the market place. The consequences of the extension of mandatory-retirement years—and possibly the total elimination of mandatory retirement—are likely to have further impact on the political outlook and behavior of the young-older persons in the population.

Advocacy

Advocacy may be broadly defined as speaking for, supporting, advising, espousing the rights of, or interceding on behalf of people before any public or private individuals, agencies, organizations, or institutions whose activities, services, plans, or policies affect or have the potential to affect the quality of life of these people.

Lowy defines advocacy as a concept borrowed from the legal profession. The advocate becomes a spokesperson for the client by presenting and arguing the client's cause when this is necessary to accomplish the objectives of the contract. The advocate is not neutral but, as in law, is a partisan spokesperson for his or her client. The advocate will engage in arguing, debating, articulation of the client's interest, bargaining, negotiating, and manipulation of the environment on behalf of the client.[9]

As was stated, the older people get, the more they have to depend on services provided by large, complex organizations—bureaucracies. Many older persons are dependent on government programs for the basic necessities of life. These programs are complicated, with a wide range of laws, regulations, rules, and procedures as well as informal practices and specific forms. Very often older people do not get their full benefits because they do not understand the program or how to use it to the greatest advantage. At other times, the system itself, because of the people directing or running it, must be pushed and prodded to provide all that it is pledged to provide under law.

The Older Americans Act Amendments of 1978 broadly mandate and set forth responsibilities that the Administration on Aging (federal), the state agency on aging (state), and the area agency on aging (local) serve as "the effective and visible advocate for the elderly."

Types of Advocacy

Advocacy may be classified according to the following types: case, legal/administrative, consumer, legislative, and systems. Case advocacy focuses on an individual's problem or situation. It may involve either internal or external advocacy activities. An information and referral service is an example of case advocacy, whereby an individual's problem or situation is discussed and the appropriate resource that should assist in alleviating the problem or improving the situation is identified.

Legal/administrative advocacy focuses on the rights of an individual or a class of individuals. Protection of rights are pursued through legal or administrative remedies. A long-term-care ombudsman program demonstrates legal/administrative internal-advocacy activities.

Consumer or citizen advocacy may be viewed as a self-help effort by a group or coalition of individuals with similar concerns and interests acting on their own behalf. Local councils on aging provide an example of consumer advocacy through external advocates.

The focus of legislative advocacy is the developing, sponsoring, supporting, and lobbying of legislation that benefits a specific population or issue. Legislative advocacy efforts may also be used to defeat the passage of legislation that has a negative or harmful effect on a specific population or issue. Advocacy for legislation may also be viewed as a strategy to effect change by both internal and external advocates.

The focus of systems advocacy is to effect a change in a system to make it more responsive to the needs of a specific population or issue. *System* may be defined as a formal arrangement or organization of policies, methods, plans, schemes, and administrative procedures. Through systems advocacy various strategies are utilized to influence or impact the system or its components by internal advocates working within and as a part of the system to bring about a change.

There are two basic forms of advocacy activities—internal and external. Internal advocates work within the system that supports them. The system may be a governmental or political structure of a human service or other service-delivery structure. Negotiation is the major mechanism utilized by internal advocates. External advocates are independent from the system in which they perform their advocacy functions. Confrontation is the major mechanism utilized by external advocates.

Case advocacy assumes a partisan stance on behalf of a person or group of people who cannot negotiate their demands alone or find redress for grievances or cut through the bureaucratic red tape. Group or class advocacy emphasizes the creation and support of neighborhood and direct-action groups representing the interests of the disadvantaged. Such advocacy is of special interest for the social worker and can be meaningful in a variety of agencies. The advocate can act as a general spokesperson for disadvantaged people and their representatives in his or her day-to-day contacts with public officials and community influentials. As a result of his or her own access to the views, plans, and informational resources of the establishment, the advocate is well equipped to provide people and groups with relevant knowledge. On the basis of training and expertise, the advocate can use such knowledge also to offer advice concerning effective methods of action for local groups. Knowing vulnerable institutional practices and the spots of maximum weakness in municipal plans and proposals, he or she often is able to suggest the most efficacious forms for direct action or other forms of pressure.

There is a danger of falling into the temptation of serving as a client's spokesperson without a clear contract with the client to do so. A lawyer does not become a spokesperson for a client until a client has retained the attorney and fully authorized him or her to perform her services. An explicit contract with the client prior to engaging in these types of advocacy activities is essential.

The need for advocacy at the agency level is frequently made evident through followup. For example, many older people who have been referred to a particular agency are not being seen by that agency for service. In followingup with individual persons, a pattern may become evident; for example the health clinic's waiting room is always full when clients arrive. Or perhaps several persons were referred to an agency that claimed to provide a home-maker service but was a companion service instead.

Legislative and system's advocacy can be effected either by citizens' groups that engage in social-action efforts (for example, the Gray Panthers) or by social agencies (for example, senior multiservice centers), by professional groups (social workers in coalition with nurses), or by governmental bodies (for example, state agencies). Joint efforts by any or all such groups presume common goals or the negotiation of conflicting interests that may mitigate against joint actions to arrive at a common front.

Advocacy by State Government

Let us review how a state governmental agency can carry out the advocacy mandate of the 1978 Amendments to the Older Americans Act. The overall goal of a state agency on aging with respect to advocacy may be stated: to effect systemic changes in social and governmental institutions to facilitate full access for elders to services, facilities, and benefits for which they may be eligible, and access to active, fulfilling and dignified lives with maximum independence, and to break down the social, economic, physical, an administrative barriers that impede such accessibility. The state agency on aging works toward this goal through its direct participation in a number of advocacy functions.

Intergovernmental Relations. Interagency cooperation is fostered by the development of ongoing working relationships with other agencies. Through intergovernmental activities, the state agency on aging represents the needs of elders with other agencies and acts to ensure that these needs are adequately reflected in the plans, programs, policies, and budgets of these agencies. The state agency on aging establishes working relationships with agencies currently administering or developing programs or services that have a direct impact on elders as well as with those agencies whose plans, policies, programs, or services have an indirect effect. It may also serve as a catalyst or facilitator for the development or coordination of programs, services, or policies that benefit elders. By working with other agencies, the state agency on aging has direct access to information that may help in identifying areas where its involvement would benefit elders.

Through a liaison role, the state agency on aging serves as an expert on elder-related issues of other agencies by providing them with technical assistance and consultation. It helps to foster an awareness and sensitivity to the needs of elders. This intergovernmental-relations function may utilize techniques ranging from informal meetings and negotiations to formal cooperative agreements. The state agency on aging may find it desirable to negotiate with other agencies for a formal sign-off policy on the plans, policies, and programs of other agencies that have an effect on elders. The development of memoranda of understanding and interagency agreements serve to formalize intergovernmental relations activities.

Planning. An advocacy function supportive of intergovernmental relations is the planning function of the state agency on aging. Through direct participation in the planning activities and processes of other agencies, the needs of elders may be represented. Through its planning linkages, the state agency on aging attempts to influence the plans, policies, programs, and budgets of other agencies so that they are responsive to the needs of elders. In the planning process, the state agency on aging identifies service gaps and priorities, facilitates program coordination and development, influences funding decisions, fosters consumer participation, and promotes mechanisms for effective monitoring and evaluation of services and plans.

A major benefit to be derived by participating in the planning processes of other agencies is access to other resources for elders. This planning involvement also facilitates coordination of the state agency on aging's plan with the plans of other agencies and helps to minimize any duplication of effort. Its own plan may be strengthened by reflecting interagency coordination. Techniques to carry out this advocacy function include negotiations, sign-off procedures, and formal interagency agreements.

State Plan Review. Through the state-plan-review function the state agency on aging determines the impact of various state plans in terms of their benefits and disbenefits for elders. The state plans that may affect elders are identified and are evaluated according to their responsiveness, quality, extent, and scope of services to be provided. State plans are also assessed with respect to the policies and priorities they may reflect. It is important to determine through the state-plan-review function what effect stated and implied policies and priorities may have on elders.

This function also provides the state agency on aging with a mechanism to evaluate the state plans of other agencies in terms of their consistency with its own state plan and its programs, policies, and priorities. Opportunities for coordination of planning, funding, and programming with other state agencies may be developed and facilitated through this review and comment process. Duplication of effort, conflicts, and lack of coordination may be dealt with through education, negotiation, and interagency agreements. This function also helps the state agency on aging to identify statewide service deficiencies and gaps that its own state-plan process must address.

Budget Review. Through budget making, state and local officials make fundamental decisions on implementing programs and policies. Through the budget-review function, the state agency on aging advocates that elders receive a fair share of resources. This function may be supportive of state plan review if the state agency on aging assumes an advocate role prior to budget requests and submissions. It may work with other agencies in budget preparation, so that the budgets reflect items that are responsive to the needs of elders.

Participation in the budget process enables the state agency on aging to present its priorities for funding of services, personnel, and facilities and to affect the system's accountability and responsiveness to the needs of elders. To assure adequate funding levels, the state agency on aging must direct its influence on the executive branch's budget, the legislative branch's appropriation, and the budget requests of individual state agencies.

Clearinghouse Review. Participation in the clearinghouse review process provides the state agency on aging with another mechanism to carry out its advocacy function. It is a procedure for coordinating federally funded programs and activities with each other and with state, regional, and local planning and program efforts. The state agency on aging has the opportunity to review the proposals of both public and private applicants seeking federal funds in relation to its own plans, programs, and priorities. The review and comment process serves as an advocacy tool as the state agency on aging evaluates proposals in terms of their effect on elders and as it attempts to maximize the potential impact of federal funds on the elder population.

Legislation/Regulation Review. The state agency on aging may effect a change or reform by utilizing the legislative or administrative rule-making mechanism. Legislation and regulations may both reflect and protect the rights and entitlements of elders. They often provide direction to plans, programs, and policies. Therefore, the state agency on aging must recognize and understand the impact and implications of both existing and proposed legislation and regulations. By evaluating and analyzing federal and state laws and regulations, the state agency on aging determines their impact on the elder population and the delivery of services, identifies any inconsistencies or conflicts with its own plans, programs, and priorities, and recognizes any implied support for its own goals and objectives. The level of involvement in undertaking this advocacy function may vary: reviewing and commenting on proposed legislation and regulations; participating in the development of legislation and regulations of other agencies; or initiating and supporting legislative and regulatory action.

If change is to be successfully effected, the most important prerequisite is the ability to recognize and identify the most appropriate points of intervention. The state agency on aging will serve as the effective and visible advocate for the elderly only if it knows when to intervene, knows which strategy to utilize, and knows how to apply its power and pressure.

The Ombudsman

Ombudsman, both as a word and as a concept, came from Sweden. The Swedish Parliament established an office of *Justiticombudsman* in 1809. This person received complaints and protected citizens from injustice, no matter where that injustice might have arisen. He was fair, impartial, and just—a citizens' defender. This office still operates in Sweden, but was almost unknown outside of the Scandanavian countries until the late 1950s. About this time many people began to feel isolated from their governments and experienced a sense of distress and distance between themselves and various administrative agencies. Within the next decade many other countries, including the United States, experimented with the ombudsman concept. In the early seventies several scandals came to light in the nursing-home industry. They shocked and horrified the American public. In response to the public clamor for government action in nursing-home reform, the president directed the Department of Health, Education and Welfare to "assist the States to establish investigative units, which would respond in a responsible and constructive way to complaints made by, or on behalf of, individuals as nursing home patients."

In December of 1971 Congress passed a supplemental appropriations act making available funds for the establishment of demonstration projects for nursing-home ombudsmen.

There were seven demonstration projects. Four of these were state-level offices linked with local units. The states were Idaho, Pennsylvania, South Carolina, and Wisconsin. A fifth control contract was awarded to the National Council of Senior Citizens to test if an ombudsman project could function independent of governmental jurisdiction. It would also test the advisability of using a national voluntary organization. The National Council of Senior Citizens chose Michigan for their demonstration project.

These five pilot programs began in June of 1972. A year later two additional states were added—Massachusetts and Oregon. These programs functioned for three years as demonstration models. At the end of the final demonstration year the commissioner on Aging invited all fifty states to submit proposals for grants to establish state offices of ombudsman.

Based on the classical ombudsman concept, the ombudsman handles citizens' complaints arising from administrative or political action by the government. The ombudsman investigates these complaints in a nonpartisan, impartial manner and attempts to persuade the parties to settle the dispute; he or she possesses no power to change or revise a judicial or administrative decision. If persuasion fails, the ombudsman may publicize unresolved grievances, reprimand officials, and recommend actions to the legislature.

The nursing-home ombudsman and patient advocate share a common purpose, the resolution of the individual patient's complaints. The patient advocate, unlike the impartial ombudsman, is a partisan who represents only the patient's interests. The advocate's primary responsibility is to assist the patient in learning about, protecting, and asserting his or her rights within the health care context. The source of the advocate's power is the patient, and therefore the advocate acts only with the consent and at the direction of the patient.

In the first stage of the grievance mechanism a patient directs his or her complaint to a resident's council, which attempts to obtain resolution of the grievance with the administrator within a stated period of time. If this effort fails, the patient or council refers the complaint to the nursing-home ombudsman, an external office established by state legislation with the powers and functions similar to those of the classical ombudsman. If the ombudsman is unable within a specified time period to resolve a meritorious grievance through negotiations with the nursing-home owner and the state inspection agency, the patient advocate receives the complaint.

The combination of the impartial ombudsman backed by the partisan advocate offers the best complement to the present system of exclusive public control over the machinery for enforcing nursing-home standards of care. Even if there is no expansion of the patient's causes of action, the combined ombudsman-advocate office gives nursing-home residents much of the protection they so need and deserve.

Social Action and Social Service Programs

In addition to politically organized people and groupings, there are an increasing number of social and service organizations that can be mobilized to advance the interests and well-being of other people, old and young, as well as to be of service to them. Community groups, civic organizations, senior centers, councils on aging, golden-age clubs, and so forth are engaged in several forms of social-action and service enterprises, although the degree, extent, and involvement varies considerably around the country. The greatest barriers to citizen involvement are usually feelings of powerlessness vis à vis complex and formidable social institutions, political mechanisms, and powerful interests in the community, as well as fear of failure and rebuff, lack of initiative, apathy, and withdrawal. However, when opportunities were made available, usually by community leaders or professionals such as social workers, and when it became feasible and manageable to organize, many thousands of older people became engaged and participated actively and competently.

The Domestic Volunteer Service Act of 1973 makes grants available to state agencies as well as to other public or nonprofit agencies to help older persons to avail themselves of opportunities for volunteer service. The following are illustrative of a series of programs presently in operation in a number of communities:

1. SERVE (Serve and Enrich Retirement by Volunteer Experience) of New York uses groups of older volunteers in state hospitals and schools for the mentally retarded. Some work with patients, some in the office, some help with other hospital duties. The group idea, both in recruitment and actual service is a major factor in the success of SERVE, because the group experience itself brings benefits to older people. They make new friendships while riding together on the bus provided for them and gain a sense of belonging and esprit de corps sharing their experiences in group discussions.

2. In the Foster Grandparent Program, older people with low incomes work with children in institutions such as schools for retarded or disturbed children, infant homes, temporary-care centers, and convalescent hospitals. "Grandparents" do not replace regular staff but establish a person-to-person relationship with a child, giving it the kind of love often missed in group-care settings. In return, "grandparents" receive an hourly stipend plus the affection and trust of the child.

3. The Green Thumb program employs low-income men and women in rural sections to beautify public areas such as parks and roadsides and to help local government and community services as aides in schools and libraries. Some provide outreach and home-maker service, make friendly visits, and provide transportation. This project is sponsored by the Farmers Union under a grant from the U.S. Department of Labor.[10] (Schools in

many parts of the country are using older volunteers as a major community resource to provide children with educational enrichment.)

4. In Illinois older members of PAM (Project for Academic Motivation) meet children in a one-to-one relationship to discuss, experiment, work with small groups, or lecture before whole classes. They work with all school ages from elementary to senior grades and with children from a wide range of income and social backgrounds. A major contribution is the revelation to many children of the link between classroom work and its future use in "the real world" outside. With AOA-demonstration-fund help the program has spread throughout Illinois and beyond through consultative help from PAM volunteers.

5. In Dade County (Florida) public schools, teacher aides are paid to perform a wide variety of noninstructional tasks that support the teacher, the pupil, and the schools in improving educational programs. Originally an AOA federally funded research and demonstration project, these teacher aides have proven so valuable that Dade County has continued to hire them as regular employees after federal funding was discontinued.

6. Under the sponsorship of the Montgomery County Federation of Women's Clubs, senior home craftsmen and good neighbor family aides in Montgomery County, Maryland, work in their own neighborhoods. In a sprawling suburban area such as this county, where extensive travel time could make part-time work prohibitive, this is important.

Senior home craftsmen are men who do minor home repairs such as replacing faucet washers, fixing locks, painting, wallpaper hanging, and other handyman jobs that are too small for commercial firms. Potential conflict with commercial businesses has been resolved by the Over-60 Counseling and Employment Service, the Washington Building Trades Council representing union members, and the Suburban Maryland Home Builders Association representing commercial contractors.

All agreed that the senior craftsmen could reasonably charge about half the going hourly rate because they would not necessarily work as fast as union members and because they might be unwilling to do everything that is required of a union workman such as heavy lifting or working high above the ground. It was also agreed that the senior craftsmen would limit themselves to small home-repair jobs that would not be profitable to commercial contractors.

There is no absolute time or dollar maximum on jobs because one homeowner might want several small jobs such as repairing screens, painting one room, or replacing stairs, which would amount to considerable time and money but would still be unprofitable to a contractor. The rule of reasonableness and a common understanding of the position of both the senior craftsmen and commercial contractors and unions govern. There have been no difficulties with this agreement.

Most of the men can do these jobs because they have had a lifetime of keeping their own homes in good repair. A few have had careers as professional carpenters or bricklayers but no longer can or want to work full-time at such strenuous jobs. One handyman teaches a home-repair course at the local YWCA to county residents who want to learn to do minor repairs themselves. The adult-education department of the public schools has also set up a class for men who want to be senior craftsmen but feel that they need some instruction.

The good neighbor family aides are women who have been home makers most of their lives and who can offer aid to other older persons or families who need help in caring for a home. The women receive training at no cost to them in the local Red Cross chapter house. A Red Cross nurse teaches home-nursing skills, the state-university extension agent teaches home economics, and a local psychiatrist who specializes in geriatrics volunteers his time to give insight on care of elderly persons. Members of the Federation provide transportation within the county to the Red Cross chapter house for the training. People from adjoining Maryland counties and the adjoining state of Virginia and the District of Columbia have also taken this training and are now working in their own communities.

The aides have had enthusiastic acceptance by the community, with the Over-60 Counseling Service receiving about twelve requests for every one it is able to fill. The Service frequently receives letters of gratitude from families who have benefited. Mothers of small children or adults who care for an elderly person in their homes are able to take short vacations knowing that their family responsibilities are in capable hands.

Although income, educational level, and social position of the aides vary widely, a study of the aides done by a graduate student shows need for additional income as most of the aides' primary reason for working. A high percentage, however, also indicated the desire to be involved in the community, to fill a real need, and to have freedom to schedule working hours as they wish.

Major Issues and Questions

Active involvement by older persons on their own behalf, as well as on behalf of others, only in its beginning stages now, will continue to expand, and it is highly possible that it will feed into the political process, particularly at the state and local levels. Professionals responsible for administrative planning and service delivery to the aging will increasingly have to recognize older persons as a constituency group with which they will need to work in partnership at all levels—community, state, and federal. The participative role of older persons in both the planning and the service-delivery processes will—in all likelihood—continue to grow along the lines stated by Estes, that is, in defining the problem, planning the strategies, and implementing the process for the development and delivery of services and facilities for the aging.[11]

To what extent will such participation enhance the participation process of the nation, as a whole? Will older people set examples to the young and counteract feelings of alienation? Will advocacy by governmental agencies reduce advocacy by citizen groups? How will the backlash response—of which Hudson speaks—be met by the organized elderly? Will "interest-group liberalism" affect the aging movement and play out its scenario as it has with other interest groups? How can "senior power" avoid the drive toward more pronounced segregation of the elderly without losing their connection with the mainstream of the population? Will public social policies toward the aged be shaped increasingly by group interests, and will these group interests become more fragmented along the young-old and old-old, along the white and nonwhite elderly, along male and female sex roles? How will future generations of aging cohorts respond to the historical moment?

Estes provides us with this challenge:

> . . . the long-range goal must be policies that provide for an adequate income, a job, decent housing, and health care; that alter the objective condition of the aged; and that change the social processes by which social policies are made and implemented in such a way that the public interests, rather than private special interests, are served. To accomplish these objectives requires the development of a comprehensive national policy on aging that does not segregate the elderly, stigmatize them or place them in a dependent and depersonalized status. To achieve such a national policy will require basic changes in our values, in our attitudes, in our behavior, and in our actions toward the elderly.[12]

Notes

1. Robert Binstock, "Interest Group Liberalism and the Politics of Aging," *Gerontologist* 2 (1972):265-280.

2. David H. Fischer, "The Politics of Aging in America, A Short History," *The Journal of the Institute of Socio-Economic Studies*, White Plains, N.Y., IV, 2, Summer 1979, 51-66.

3. Ibid.

4. Gray Panthers, "Statement of Purpose," Philadelphia, Pennsylvania, 1970.

5. Legislative Council for Older Americans "Statement," Boston, Massachusetts, 1972.

6. Robert Binstock, "Aging and the Future of American Politics," *Annals of the American Academy of Polit. Soc. Sci.* 415 (1974):199-212.

7. R. Hudson, "The Graying of the Federal Budget and Its Consequences for Old Age Policy," *The Gerontologist*, Pt. I, Vol. 18, No. 5, Oct. 1978, 428-440.

8. Ibid.

9. Louis Lowy, *Social Work with the Aging*, New York, Harper & Row, 1979, p. 228.

10. U.S. Department of Health, Education and Welfare, *Let's End Isolation*, DHEW Publication (OHDS) 78-20129 (Washington, D.C., 1973).

11. Carroll L. Estes, *The Aging Enterprise* (San Francisco: Jossey-Bass, 1979).

12. Ibid., p. 247.

**Social Policies:
Planning for Tomorrow**

Public social policies define courses of action to be followed by the appropriate groups within the government. These policies are based on assumptions and are directed at specific concerns, problems, or issues.

The changing demographic and political realities express themselves in continual assessment of public policies toward the aged. The services and income strategy that public policy has designed are likely to come under scrutiny. Answers must be found for such issues as: how to insure that our system of support responds effectively to widely varying circumstances of the elderly and their families; how to make certain that the efforts of government at any level actually enhance and add to the compassionate care and support of families for their elders, how to halt the fragmentation, waste, and duplication that have come with the great proliferation of programs for the elderly at every level of government. Other issues include: how to achieve a simplification of rules and regulations that have erected barriers for older people rather than opened up opportunities for them; how to build partnership with state and local governments to improve the management and delivery of service to the well elderly and to the chronically impaired; how to ensure that federally supported programs do not upset existing services for the elderly, especially those in the voluntary sector and those existing in the informal network provided by families, friends, and neighbors as has been amply documented.

There is already evidence that the entrance of federal programs into the community causes the exit of other programs or volunteer efforts. How can we build incentives into our system of care that would encourage appropriate responses in each case? How can we guarantee the right of elderly citizens to choose their own alternatives? By what mechanisms shall individual needs be measured or provider services be created? These are just some of the few questions that come with increasing bureaucratization of what Carroll Estes calls "the aging enterprise." In her view, politics, economics, and social structure have far more to do with the aging process than the biological and physiological changes that occur in the later years of life: "These two ideologies, separatism and pluralism, are at the core of American social policy for the aged."[1] They have had a major effect on public programs. She points out that the various programs, such as social security, medicare, medicaid, food stamps, housing, Title XX, social services, and the Older Americans Act itself have not met the needs of the elderly, since "the policies are largely symbolic and reflect dominant perspectives about the aged. They tend to segregate the aged, often with the poor, as a special class in society."[2] She goes on to say: "The Older Americans Act reflected the growing visibility of interest groups for the elderly and the awakening of academic, recreational and social work professionals to a new field of work."[3] During the economic crises of the 1970s, funding for services was shifted from the federal level to the decentralized network of state units and area agencies on aging, under the Nixonian "new federalism." By assigning these agencies responsibility to look for local resources, coupled with diminished federal financial handouts, it was hoped that the growth of federal economic commitments could be minimized. In the late 1970s, the policies began to shift again, abandoning the conception of the social definition of the problems of the aged, and viewing them as an at-risk population whose individual members have diminished capacities that need shoring up. Where are we going in the 1980s and 1990s?

Some Trends and Policy Questions for the Future

The elderly population will be older in 1990 than it is today with an additional 7 percent aged 75 and older than in 1977; more elderly will be women, the proportion over the next decade rising from 59.4 percent in 1977 to 61.7 percent; more elderly people will be married, especially those over 75. The percentage of married elderly will swell from 38.6 percent in 1977 to 43.5 in 1990; more elderly women will have grown children. Seventy percent of those aged 65 to 74 will have two or more adult children as compared with 57 percent in 1977.[4] The most important trend is the rapid rate at which the elderly population is expanding, particularly its older-older sector.

Between 1977 and 2035, the total population in the United States is projected to grow by about 40 percent, from 217 million to 304 million persons. The elderly population is projected to more than double in size during this same period from 33 to 71 million persons. The segments of the elderly population that will be growing most rapidly will be the oldest of the old and women and persons of races other than white, the same groups that have suffered more from such common problems of the elderly as poor health, social isolation, and poverty.

The population 75 years of age and older has experienced a tenfold increase since 1900, the age group 85 and older has grown by about seventeen times, and the size of the 60-and-over population has increased by nearly seven times. Currently, about nearly 40 percent of the elderly population is 75 and over, and this proportion is expected to increase to 45 percent by the year 2000. The 85-and-older group now constitutes one of every sixteen elderly persons; by 2000 they will represent one of every eleven.[5]

Successive generations of elders will be better educated and if not more financially well off at retirement at least will have lived a more affluent life than their predecessors. Three factors important for social policy emerge from these trends: The new generations of elders because of their educational and financial backgrounds will have greater expectations for services. This group will undoubtedly be seeking different types of services and may come with greater political ability to be effective in gaining what they seek. However, because of the increasing numbers of elders, the demand for existing services will at least stay the same if not increase with the increasing elderly population. As a result, the range of services will expand rather than simply shift in response to new demands.

The second factor is the economic status of succeeding generations of the elderly. Pension plans and the level of benefits will be increased over those available to the elderly of today, but these increases will probably be lost to increasing costs of energy, food, and housing. As is presently the case, the level of benefits is largely fixed at the time of retirement, so that older cohorts of elders, because of inflation, will have smaller resource bases as their need for support increases.

The third factor relates to the ratio of active workers to retired citizens that will change dramatically over the future from six to one today to three to one in 2030. This ratio is important because it suggests how many active workers are available to support programs for the elderly. We can estimate this ratio by comparing the number of citizens 65 and over to those 20 to 64. This is rather imprecise, since some persons over 65 are not retired, and many people age 20 to 64 are not workers. But the historical changes in this ratio are extraordinary nonetheless: in 1940 there were nine citizens age 20 to 64 for every citizen 65 or over; today it is six to one; by 2030, it will be only three to one.

At this date these projections may vary somewhat, as the long-term effects of changes in mandatory-retirement policies cannot be assessed as yet.

At present, we have two distinct conceptions of retirement: The first is support for workers who have reached old age and can no longer work. The second, more recent conception views retirement as a reward not necessarily related to old age: simply a reward for a certain period of work. In the armed forces, for example, a pension is available after twenty years of service, regardless of age; workers in the federal civil service, and in many state and local governments, can retire on full pension at age 55 with thirty years of service.

New retirement policies will have to be considered; for example different kinds of work arrangements that can accommodate greater numbers of older people in the work force, such as phased retirement and increased part-time work. Several studies suggest that as many as four out of five workers would prefer to reduce their years of retirement and redistribute more leisure in the middle years of life; this highlights the need for more flexible career patterns.[6] New kinds of incentives will have to be reviewed like those provided in the 1977 social security amendments, which increase a worker's retirement benefits by 3 percent each year of work past 65. Many countries in the industrialized world are already exploring these options.

How Can Better Income Security Be Provided?

The social security system dominates income provision. Unlike most employer pension plans, it covers nearly the entire population and even in times of galloping inflation it still provides more protection against inflation than existing pension plans or savings. And yet about one-quarter of the elderly are either poor or "near poor," that is, their incomes are less than 125 percent of the poverty line.

Social security does not operate in isolation. In 1977 supplemental-security income reached 2.3 million aged beneficiaries, about 70 percent of whom also received social security. There are sixty-eight different retirement plans in the federal government; more than six thousand state and local pension plans, and thousands of private plans. Jointly, they pay out close to $50 billion in benefits. Of all new social security retirees, 50 percent have additional pension income. Tax breaks accorded to pension plans and social security income, and to elderly taxpayers, total more than $21 billion in 1980. Finally, there are private savings, which provide an estimated $15 to 20 billion in income for retirees.[7]

These income-support programs leave us caught between two conflicting pressures with regard to our income policy for older people: the pressure to keep future costs under control and the pressure to increase benefits to persons whose income is inadequate absolutely and relatively. Resolving this problem depends, in part, on the total amount that society is willing to commit for income maintenance. But it depends, as well, on integrating this patchwork of systems more effectively and managing the resources we do provide so that they do the most good. A basic question, then, is what the ratio should be between income earned before retirement and income thereafter. But beyond this lie questions of how the overall system treats those at the top—and at the bottom—of the scale. Social security benefits are exempt from taxes. It seems at least open to discussion whether a wealthy lawyer, doctor, or business executive with a $50,000 pension should receive social security benefits free from any obligation to pay taxes. At the other end of the scale, we have to consider the plight of those for whom social security benefits are the sole source of income, whose earning record may not entitle them to the greatest amount. And taxing social security would constitute double taxation and would hardly be equitable in relation to the total society.

Is supplemental-security income, which focuses income only on those at the low end of the income scale, a more efficient method? How do we compare the value of efficiency and the resources it frees for serving unmet needs at the price of a stigmatized "means-test" against the social security system that brings a certain degree of minimal economic independence to many people who would otherwise be poor, and does so with no means test? Targeting limited resources to those in greatest need is a major policy issue that haunts many a welfare state around the world today, notably England, Sweden, and France.[8]

Another critical question is the relationship between private and public pensions. Private pensions have spread such that they now cover about 45 percent of the work force, but that growth was in a period when persistent inflation did not exist. Even if inflation rates were cut in half, it would still call into question their ability over time to provide benefits that will keep pace with price increases. If private pension plans appear unlikely to assume a major role in providing retirement income, do we wish to continue to encourage the creation of this layer on top of social security? At present, we do just that, by providing substantial tax benefits for contributions to pension plans. And the Employment Retirement Income Security Act (ERISA) has not fulfilled its promise, nor is it likely to be able to alleviate its continuing difficulties, as witnessed by congressional concerns.[9]

How Shall Health and Social
Services Policies Be Directed?

Between now and the year 2025, it is estimated that expenses for persons over 65 under the present medicare and medicaid programs will increase, in real terms, more than ten times, twice as fast a pace as the increases in social security. The inflation that these figures reflect is especially harsh on the elderly, given their great needs and their overriding reliance on fixed incomes. Containment of health costs is certainly an urgent necessity; the question as to the "how" produces tension and conflicts among health care providers and few solutions are in sight.

We should be concerned about costs, but we must be even more concerned about the shortcomings and deficiencies of this expensive system. For all the money we spend, major health needs of the population in the nation remain unmet. As the elderly population increases, especially those 75 and older, who are likely to have more serious health problems, these needs will increase. Even with medicaid and medicare, many older people must pay large amounts out of pocket to meet these needs today. In 1976, these expenses averaged over $400, virtually the same in real terms as they paid out of pocket before medicare and medicaid arrived.

A rational, comprehensive, efficient, caring, and humane system for delivering health and social services would include: adequate, supervised residential facilities for those who lack families but want to live in their communities; special services for those who live at home but need help from outside: transportation or shopping assistance, help with meals and personal care; a range of alternative options between the hospital and the nursing home, including home-health care and day-care programs; innovative and compassionate ways of caring for the terminally ill outside the traditional hospital or nursing home in or through hospices. Because of our medical emphasis on short-term cure rather than on long-term care we have not developed an adequate system of community and home-health care. In Sweden, there is one home health aide for every 120 people; in this country, one for every 5,000.[10]

Although a social services strategy is being advocated as an equal partner to a health approach, the problems of inadequacy, poor delivery mechanisms, and confusing philosophies and policies in the social service field must be acknowledged. There is also increasing conflict about whether to give priority to all the elderly or to poor, minority, and impaired older persons. Another dilemma is the very philosophy behind the enactment of the Older Americans Act, namely, that the elderly do not get their fair share when they are "mainstreamed" with other ages. When HEW Secretary Califano testified in the House on the 1978 amendments to the act, he advised deferring any substantive changes in the act while working on some of these problems. He said:

> Over the past two decades, Federal, State and local agencies have rapidly expanded these programs to serve older people. But our compassion has too often exceeded our understanding. We have created a virtual maze which is often incomprehensible to the older people we are supposed to serve. Now we must take the time to re-examine carefully the organization and delivery of our services if they are to meet the pressing needs of the next decade.[11]

Mental health policies need to be coordinated with physical health policies. It is important to note basic differences between health and social models. Health care is essentially dependency-creating because its complicated technologies require a great deal of decision making by the technicians, primarily the physician as the manager of health care, and not only medical care, in the present schema of things. The use of health technology is costly, and a major way to limit its cost is to avoid its use except for purely medical care.

What many believe to be the core of social practice is mutual aid modeled after the caring, nurturing, and coping roles of the family itself. In the social model every attempt is made to strengthen existing and available care within the family, only turning to the development of familylike supports when the real thing is not available or cannot do the whole job. Although there has been an increase in the last ten years in federal monies for social services for the elderly, both through age-integrated programs made possible by Title XX of the Social Security Act and age-segregated programs of the Older Americans Act, there is still hesitation about just how far government should get involved in functions that many citizens believe to be the province of the family or at least of voluntary services. The limitations of an income strategy are being increasingly appreciated and understood, particularly for the frail elderly and their families who, even with money, cannot cope with problems of daily living, and the call for a combined income and service strategy gets louder.

Beyond developing the right kinds of health and social services, there is the problem of making them readily accessible and acceptable. At present, an older person faces a bewildering maze that must be negotiated even to learn what services are available, much less to obtain the right kind and mix. How can we end the fragmentation of services for the elderly? How can we ensure that the needs of the elderly are properly identified and get the care they need? Inspired by a concern for effective and economic management of social programs is the importance of coordinated and integrated services. Such an emphasis is particularly important for the elderly with their multiple and changing service needs. Although coordination implies a mechanism that will link an individual with the various resources in the community through knowledge of what exists and how it might be obtained, integration implies a concentration of services within agencies. The result of this type of concentration may result in an actual loss in range and variety of service availability and perhaps limited access to services, either through a restriction in the number of entry points to the service system or through more stringent eligibility or entrance requirements. Do premature integration and coordination of services lead to inadequate development of resources because such efficiency within the service system does not allow individuals enough opportunities to enter the system and receive the services they need? Or is the single entry the most desirable approach, since it facilitates the accessability and useability of all necessary services? A long-term-care demonstration project of a channeling-type agency, TRIAGE, has been evaluated to assess its viability and effectiveness. It tested the concept of single-entry and single-billing systems for health and social service needs of the elderly. The report showed improvement of morale and health, and 25 to 30 percent avoided institutionalization through use of home care and other services and cost savings.[12]

How can a continuum of physical, mental, and social services be erected that takes into account changing needs of an older population over time and the constraints of fiscal resources in competition with other societal priorities in the social and nonsocial sector? How can easy movement between components of care be encouraged—those of prevention, preventive interventions, community care, ambulatory treatment, and institutional care? How can a national health insurance system be created that offers such a continuum and has the capacity to provide these services to young, middle-aged, and older people? It requires enormous fiscal, organizational ingenuity, and political acumen to accomplish this feat!

As we seek to improve the delivery of health and social services, we must not forget the critical role of research. We need to learn more about the diseases that afflict the elderly and how these diseases can be treated most effectively or prevented in the first place. We need to learn more about the way coordinated programs and services work and how they improve the quality of life.

The term *quality of life*, which originated in France and has gradually entered the lexicon of America, applies to the aging as well as to any other age group. Life-long education, especially during the leisure years, does enhance mental and physical well-being. In addition, the opportunity to acquire new skills and knowledge becomes important for older people to cope with societal and technological changes, to prepare for reemployment if so desired, and to remain actively engaged in the affairs of state. To date, however, government has generally ignored the older adult learner. Less than 1 percent of the $14 billion the federal government spends on education for educating persons past compulsory school age is allocated for persons 45 and over. The Higher Education Act's life-long learning provisions need to be strengthened and appropriate funding made available to implement them; life-long learning should be redirected into work- and retirement-related areas, but any new adult-learner program should be coordinated with resources that already exist. To illustrate: During 1978-1979 the DeCordova Museum School of Art in Lincoln, Massachusetts, in cooperation with the Acton, Concord, Lincoln, Stow, and Maynard councils on aging, conducted an outreach program for the low-income elderly. This program, funded by the National Endowment for the Arts and Title III of the Older Americans Act, integrated fifty senior citizens into regularly scheduled art classes, which normally serve a younger and much more affluent population. This program demonstrated that the elderly want and can successfully participate in substantial educational programs if the psychological, financial, and physical barriers to their participation are removed.

It was shown that the elderly do want to learn, that they can benefit from participation in a high-quality educational program that stimulates their mental growth and that participation in stimulating activities can indeed improve or prevent the deterioration of mental and/or physical health and aid in a healthy adaptation to old age. Participants in this program have commented that the DeCordova project has allowed them "to do something that I never thought I could do," "to meet new people," "a chance to get out and make new friends," "to learn the pleasure of creating," and to "develop a new sense of accomplishment." The teachers have commented that the elderly students show tremendous interest and at times even learn at rates much faster than our regular student body.[13]

To help assure the elderly of the equality of education opportunities, financial assistance should be made readily available to them. At the present time, education money in gerontology is mostly used to educate and train service providers. Virtually none is allocated to preventive education to help the elderly care for themselves or to training programs that would help them remain active in society. The training needs of those providing services to the elderly will increase; however, what is also needed is to look at public policy regarding education for older adults.

What Directions Should Housing Policies Take?

Testifying before the House Select Committee on Aging in 1977, Monsignor Charles Fahey, in his role as president of the American Association of Homes for the Aging, urged public-housing policy that would be more realistic in regard to the social needs of those who live in federally assisted housing projects:

> The single social change we could make affecting the lives of the elderly, that would promote the greatest social benefit for the least number of dollars would be to take all the federally-assisted housing, whether public housing or 202 or 236, and build into the basic financing mechanisms—the operational financing mechanism—a certain floor of soft management services, and recognize this as an integral part of the subsidy, an integral part of the rent. I am not talking about all social services but I am talking about certain fundamental, soft management services: the ability to know the person in the facility, the ability to create a positive interaction among the people in the facility, the ability of the facility to create linkages with the community and serve as advocate for those individuals to get community services of whatever sort, certain nutritional counseling services, and certain public health type services.[14]

How can various options in living arrangements be realized, given the changing nature of our elderly population, from assisting people with maintaining their private homes, (if they so desire), to arranging for supportive living environments, such as foster home care, family care homes, community residents, congregate housing, group residences, retirement communities? How will supports be made available to rural elderly who are often geographically isolated and have limited access to services? What programs will facilitate mobility and insure physical safety to make "a home really a home?" Of particular import for the future will be the way in which the special needs of aged are being addressed, and issues of double as well as triple jeopardy are being dealt with. Can we plan for a new generation of elderly who will be specially assisted to overcome discriminatory barriers, because of race, sex, or ethnicity? How will they be integrated into the mainstream of the older population? Will their special needs of today become special assets of tomorrow? How will their cultural and ethnic backgrounds be utilized to enrich their own lives and those of others? How will the natural (informal) network be linked with the formal service bureaucracy and become an integrative force in the lives of the American community?

Families provide a wide range of services, from escorting the elderly on trips and helping with shopping and household chores to more complicated health and rehabilitative care. Yet it is also true that the extended family living in a single household is no longer so common. Of persons 65 and over with living children, 36 percent lived with their children twenty years ago; by 1975, that percentage had fallen to 18 percent. So far we have designed our programs for the elderly only with the individual in mind, not the family unit. Our programs for financing chronic care do little to permit and encourage home-care administered by family members, unlike countries such as Sweden, Norway, Denmark, and West Germany.

We need to establish programs that help families care for their aged members. We cannot expect all doctors, nurses, social workers, or bureaucrats to be as sensitive in meeting the needs of the elderly as a child or grandchild, brother or sister, even though many do their very best to be empathetic and to combine their head with their heart.

Because families themselves are so various, our approaches must also be varied: For those who do live with relatives, for example, day-care or respite service should be available, to give the caring relative the freedom to leave home without worrying about the aged person, a service of growing importance as the proportion of women in the work force increases.

For the majority of the elderly who live on their own, either in couples or singly, we need other kinds of services; supervised residential arrangements that will permit them to remain in the community where the family can more easily support them. And for those who lack families nearby, we must think of developing surrogates, people who volunteer, or are trained, to give the same kind of comfort, and show the same kind of concern, as family members; who can provide the individualized and personal attention for which there is no substitute.

Two policy issues can be identified here: (1) what alternative services can be developed to enhance, at least in part, the role of the family, and (2) what are the consequences of various programs for the elderly on the nature and structure of their families? Building on these questions, we may further ask: What are the unintended consequences of the services provided for individuals and their families? In the attempt to provide for the immediate fulfillment of a presumed need, planners often do not consider what the unintended results of a program might be and whether they are positive or negative. These unintended consequences might include increased dependency as a result of participation, increased socializing or access to other services, accentuation of shifts in family relations that inhibit informal delivery of social services, or increased demand for services through increased social and emotional dependency or through increased expectations. Once a program is in operation, this question becomes one of whether the program is fulfilling its expectations through providing the intended services or reaching the intended group of people. Basically, the answer to this question can be found in three types of research: needs assessment, social-impact analysis, and functional program evaluation. Such research provides information necessary to the development of social policy because it helps to insure, although not guarantee, that appropriate programs are developed to fill real needs, that such programs do not produce unintended negative consequences (iatrogenic effects), and that resources are used more effectively by services being delivered to the people intended to receive their benefit.

Training

The design of policies and the planning of programs and services are predicated on the availability of competent, committed, and compassionate professionals, paraprofessionals, and volunteers. For this reason the existence of adequately conceived, designed, and implemented training programs are a sine qua non in the mosaic of social policies for the aging. Development of an adequate supply of trained personnel to meet the nationwide needs of the elderly is dependent on coordinated planning, programming, and appropriate funding at the federal level to ensure that this occurs. A training program, national in scope and federally coordinated, must address and seek to correct past deficiencies in training that currently impede effective service delivery and research investigations; future capacity to assure an ongoing supply of competent personnel must be developed, and barriers to service that stem from misunderstanding and prejudice toward the elderly must be removed.

The phasing and priorities of training and the establishment of guidelines for new manpower development should be formed by a careful analysis of current and projected service needs in relation to existing manpower supply and deployment, which has been sadly lacking so far. Training efforts are to be directed to facilities in colleges and universities, existing service providers, paid and volunteer policy planners and shapers, current students in educational institutions, and particularly those who need and want to update their knowledge and skills in continuing education programs.

Concluding Thoughts

All societies respond in some way to the increased dependencies of their older members. In the past, societal responses have ranged from a harsh survival-of-the-fittest strategy to a more humane strategy of family responsibility for care of the aged. Modern industrial societies have emphasized family responsibility and have provided bureaucratically organized health and social services for the elderly. This shift from informal family to formal service agency is seen as a response both to the increasing numbers of older persons in modern societies and to the changing characteristics of modern families, which make caring for their own members difficult.

It has been stressed that an understanding of services to the elderly requires that social interests other than those of elderly service recipients must also be considered. The middle-aged children of aging parents are freed of much of their responsibility for the daily care of those parents. These middle-aged workers are thus freer to meet the demands of an economy that increasingly requires mobility and that both husband and wife be employed. Formal social services make it easier for adult children to attain filial maturity. This is an ability to freely give support and comfort to their parents without depriving those parents of their identities and making them dependent.[15]

These same middle-aged workers are also responsible for payment of taxes to fund services. The taxpayer's revolt of the late seventies is a major force against expenditure of public funds for all kinds of community services to the aged. Problems of aging are the domain of the individual and the family, argue the conservatives, and not the concern of government. The position of leaders of the taxpayer's revolt is thus not unlike the position of the Social Darwinists. Conservatives such as Milton Friedman stress that the real interests of the taxpayer and the society as a whole are best met by cutting taxes and cutting governmentally provided community services to the bare minimum and instead make them available through the mechanism of the "free market." However, it appears that, at least for those who are old or who have aging parents, this is a questionable assumption. An international study of community services for the aged indicated that most services are used by the fastest growing group of old people, those over 75.[16]

The middle-aged family that votes for reduced taxes may also be voting for no assistance in meeting the needs of their aging parents. If community services for the aged are not available, or out of financial reach of individuals, then the choice is often between total care by the family or total institutionalization in a nursing home. Thus one major concern is that if governmentally financed community services for the aged and aging are not available, and on a substantially larger scale than is even presently the case, then the quality of life will continue to be poor for a great many persons. (It is quite unrealistic to expect that the private sector will create a service system that is available to the average older citizen any more than private schools are the answer to meeting the educational needs of our younger population.) On the other hand, if services are provided on a larger scale, then we run the risk that the bureaucracies created will become self-serving institutions, or worse yet, agencies for social control of the aged. We must, then, both provide the needed services and humanize the bureaucracy. Humanizing the bureaucracy is quite different than making it just accountable. The former asks that it be responsive to clients, the latter that it be responsive to politicians and bureaucrats.

Late in 1978, the General Assembly of the United Nations approved a resolution directing its secetary-general to organize a world assembly on the elderly to be conducted in 1982. However, action on designating 1982 as a world year on aging was postponed. A proposal for a world assembly on aging and a world year on aging had been made to the UN General Assembly several years earlier by Senator Frank Church, then chairman of the U.S. Senate Special Commitee on Aging. After the House of Representatives' Select Committee on Aging was established, its chairman, Congressman Claude Pepper, obtained House approval of a supporting resolution. During the time that it was being considered, the Church-Pepper proposal received strong support from the U.S. delegation to the General Assembly, encouraged by HEW's International Office, working in conjunction with the Department of State. Final approval of the proposed resolution was supported by both developing and developed member nations.

The UN resolution calls for "a World Assembly on the Elderly in 1982, a forum to launch an international action programme aimed at guaranteeing economic and social security to older persons, as well as opportunities to contribute to community development." Pursuant to this resolution, the secretary-general requested all member nations to submit suggestions for "a draft programme . . . and recommendations on the organization and objectives of the World Assembly." Following a canvass of the principal federal agencies and voluntary organizations identified with the aging field, HEW, with the collaboration of the Department of State, submitted a statement of U.S. recommendations in response to the secretary-general's request.

The statement proposes that the designated assembly participants include political leaders, government and nongovernment specialists, and concerned citizens, including the elderly, who would address four technical and four general areas related to the assembly's expressed purpose as set forth in the resolution. The four technical areas suggested are: the place and contributions of older people in society; maintenance of income in the later years; health, medical care, and rehabilitation; and family relationships, housing, living arrangements, and community services. The general areas proposed are: awareness, attitudes, and rights of the elderly; government organization and policy development; information and counseling services; and research and training policies and practices. Currently, the UN General Assembly is engaged in selecting a secretary-general for the world assembly on the elderly and is developing a plan for it.[17]

The Elderly as a Resource

Too often we have looked at the older population as one in need of support rather than as a group that has a great deal to contribute to themselves and others. As consumers and as producers of goods and services, they constitute an economic resource. In the political arena they are exercising their political responsibilities as vital and active citizens. In the social sphere, they act as providers of services, as professionals, paraprofessionals, and as volunteers in many programs that link the old with the old and the old with the young. In educational programs, from kindergarten to postdoctoral programs, in private and public institutions, older adults, as learners and teachers, act as examples and communicate their life experiences, "their wisdom as well as their follies," gained in having lived sixty, seventy, or eighty years.

As a psychological resource, in what Butler calls "elder functions," they transmit values and traditions of the society to subsequent generations and act as role models for the young by teaching them how to grow older and by making positive use of that stage of life, with dignity and integrity that makes each life-cycle unique, worthwhile, and meaningful.[18]

Supervaluation of youth, stereotypes, fear of aging, and many myths about the aging person present the biggest problems for the older adult. Despite statistical assertion, priorities are not accorded the elderly, and older adults themselves, at least the current generation, are reluctant to seek out or accept services because they view them as charity rather than as entitlements.

It is anticipated that future generations will be more oriented to using publicly provided services as a matter of right for past efforts and for the amount of money paid into the economy prior to voluntary or mandatory retirement:

Despite the uncertainties of the present and the future, responses to the facts of an aging population and the specialized needs of the young-middle and the old-old will continue to occur and expand. As the special needs for locomotion and mobility of the aging are reflected in environmental design, transportation systems, and communication networks, and as alternatives to support the individual indentities of older persons continue to be recognized and developed, particularly at the neighborhood and community levels, changes will occur in the fundamental organization and delivery of services. Community health systems, combining environmental, social, health, education, and recreational needs will increasingly come together in new organizational forms which will respond to the multi-dimensional needs of the older persons through interdisciplinary linkages. Special issues in regard to the centralization of planning and administration and the decentralization of services will occur. Through such approaches, hopefully, life, as well as death for older persons will increase in dignity and meaning.[19]

And, hopefully, life and death—as part of life—will increase in dignity and meaning for everybody in our society—young and old and those in the middle—to assure a common bond and an affinity with each other—to answer the biblical question "Am I my brother's keeper?" with "I am my brother's brother" or "I am my sister's sister" at any time in the journey throughout our lives. To move toward this goal is truly the human quest, the Olympian and Faustian adventure that does make life and living worthwhile!

Notes

1. Carroll L. Estes, *The Aging Enterprise* (San Francisco: Jossey-Bass, 1979), p. 4.

2. Ibid., p. 223.

3. Ibid., pp. 223-224.

4. Richard Wertheimer and Sheila Zedlewski, *Older American Reports*, 9 January 1980, p. 3.

5. U.S. Department of Health, Education and Welfare, Federal Council on Aging, *Public Policy and the Frail Elderly*, DHEW Publication (OHDS) 79-20959 (Washington, D.C., 1978).

6. Max Kaplan, *Leisure: Lifestyle and Lifespan* (Philadelphia: W.B. Saunders, 1979).

7. James H. Schulz, "The Economic Impact of an Aging Population," *Gerontologist* 13 (1973):111-117.

8. U.S. Social Security Administration, *Social Security Programs Throughout the World*, Office of Research and Statistics Research Report no. 44 (Washington, D.C.: U.S. Government Printing Office, 1973).

9. Pension Policy Commission Act (PL 96-14) extends through 24 May 1981 the President's Commission on Pension Policy, which is reviewing

public and private retirement, survivor and disability programs, in terms of gaps in coverage, appropriate retirement ages, and financial solvency.

10. Virginia Little, "Open Care for the Aging" *Aging* (U.S. Dept. of HEW, Admin. on Aging) November/December 1979, p. 7.

11. HEW Secretary Califano, testimony to U.S. House of Representatives in 1978.

12. *Aging Services News*, Bethesda, Md., no. 68 (28 February 1980): p. 3.

13. Report by DeCordova Museum School of Art, Lincoln, Mass., 1979.

14. Charles J. Fahey, "Who Is Old?" testimony at House Select Committee on Aging, 1977.

15. Louis Lowy, "Adult Children and Their Parents: Dependency or Dependability," *Long Term Care and Health Services Administration Quarterly* (Fall 1977):245.

16. Sheila Kamerman, "Community Services for the Aged: The View from Eight Countries," *The Gerontologist* 16, vol. 3, 1976, p. 537.

17. *Aging*, AOA Publication, February 1980, p. 2.

18. Robert H. Butler, *Why Survive? Being Old in America* (New York: Harper and Row, 1975).

19. Walter M. Beattie, Jr., "Aging and the Social Services," in Robert H. Binstock and Ethel Shanas, eds., *Handbook of Aging and the Social Sciences* (New York: Van Nostrand, Rheinhold, 1976), p. 641.

Appendix A:
Structure and Function
of the U.S. Government

Government in the United States functions at three levels: federal, state, and local. Each of these three levels of government has three separate or independent branches: (1) the legislative branch, which makes or passes laws; (2) the executive branch, which carries out these laws; and (3) the judicial branch, which interprets the laws. These three branches of the federal government were created by the U.S. Constitution. The structure, function, and procedures of each branch of government follow.

The Legislative Branch

Functions

The legislative is a branch of government that has primary responsibility for creating or enacting laws. At the federal level, the legislative branch is called Congress; at the state level, the branch is usually called the state legislature; for example, the California State Legislature; and at the local level, the branch is often called the city council or the county board of supervisors. The laws passed by Congress and by the state legislatures are called statutes. An example of a federal statute affecting the elderly is the Older Americans Act. An example of a state statute affecting the elderly is a state hearing-aid-dealers-licensure statute. The laws passed by city councils or by county boards of supervisors are often called ordinances. For instance, the city council might enact an ordinance providing for property-tax relief for elderly homeowners.

The U.S. Congress has other important functions in addition to lawmaking. First is "legislative oversight"—to assure itself that the executive branch is administering the laws the way Congress intended, various congressional committees scrutinize the operations of the hundreds of governmental programs. For instance, appropriate committees may examine the Administration on Aging, in the Departments of Health and Human Services and Education to determine whether it is thoroughly carrying out the mandates of the Older Americans Act. Closely related to the oversight function is the appropriation function; Congress must appropriate all money that the government spends. If it is unhappy with a specific program, Congress may reduce or eliminate the appropriation for that program.

Based on material by Max J. Skidmore and Marshall C. Wanke.

Third, a function of individual legislators is offering services to the constituents in their district. Thus, an older person may write to his congressman complaining that his SSI check has suddenly, inexplicably been cut. The congressman's office may call over to the proper office in the Social Security Administration and straighten the matter out.

A fourth function of Congress is conducting investigations, debates, and hearings and otherwise contributing to public information. A good example concerning the elderly would be the many public hearings held by the Senate Special Committee on Aging on subjects including: criminal victimization to health care, nutrition, transportation, and social services.

A fifth legislative function, limited to the Senate, is participation in the selection of appointive officials. Article II, Section 2 of the U.S. Constitution requires that the Senate give its "advice and consent" before the president may appoint the major offices of government.

Structure and Organization

The U.S. Congress, as well as most state legislatures, are bicameral—they consist of two houses, usually a house and a senate. The U.S. House consists of congressmen who are apportioned among the states according to population. It has at least one member from each state, with a total membership of 435 (1980). Each congressman serves for two years, and then may be reelected. The U.S. Senate has 100 senators, each state having two members. Each senator serves a six-year term.

The real work of Congress is done in the committees. To achieve greater efficiency in handling the overwhelming number of bills, Congress has provided for committees to divide up the labor and permit a certain degree of specialization. There are four kinds of committees: select (ad-hoc bodies created for a specific purpose); joint (composed of members of both houses); conference (used to settle differences between the two houses whenever one passes a bill not identical to the same bill passed by the other house); and standing (the heart of the committee system—permanent units to consider proposed legislation and recommend action). There are several committees in Congress that are concerned specifically with the needs of older persons. Examples include the Senate Special Committee on Aging, the House Select Committee on Aging, and the Senate Subcommittee on Aging of the Labor and Public Welfare Committee.

Procedures

The path of a bill is quite long and arduous: (1) It may be introduced by congressmen in the House. (2) It is referred to the appropriate committee, and then to the subcommittee with jurisdiction over the subject matter involved. (3) The subcommittee may hold hearings. (4) If it recommends the bill favorably, the committee may report it favorably. If the committee does not, it usually dies. (5) The committee may add amendments of its own or rewrite the bill. (6) The bill will then be placed on a calendar and must be cleared through the Rules Committee. (7) If the Rules Committee acts favorably, the measure goes before the full House for debate and parliamentary maneuvering. (8) If the bill receives a favorable vote, it goes to the Senate. (9) Meanwhile, or afterwards, a similar procedure may be carried out in the Senate. (10) If the House and Senate bills differ, a conference committee meets to iron out the differences. (11) The bill becomes an act of Congress and goes to the president to sign into law or to veto. It is obvious that there are many pitfalls along the way. And if the bill survives, money must still be appropriated.

The Executive Branch

The executive branch seeks to implement and enforce the laws made by the legislative branch. The executive branch may be divided into two parts: the elected leader and his policy subordinates under his or her direct control; and the bureaucracies, controlled by civil service hiring. Although the public may think of the president, the governor, or the mayor when the executive is mentioned, the bureaucracy is the only part of the system with which most persons will have any personal contact—the internal revenue agent, the post office clerk, the SSA employee.

As head of the executive branch, the president is the head of the entire federal bureaucracy. He determines priorities, suggests legislation, vetos legislation he does not favor, presides over the budgetary process (with the assistance of the Office of Management and Budget), and issues executive orders. An executive order is a directive issued under the authority of the president, either by him personally or by one of the executive departments. Executive orders usually involve a change in the regulations of an agency or an action that must be taken to implement legislation.

The office of the governor, at the state level, strongly resembles that of a miniature presidency, with some exceptions. The typical governor faces greater constitutional restrictions than the president and must often share executive authority with other elected officials such as the attorney general, secretary of state, or auditor.

The bureaucracies, at both the federal and state levels, are large. Today, in the federal government, there are twelve departments whose heads constitute the Cabinet. Particularly important to the elderly are the Department of Health, Education and Welfare (now the Department of Health and

Human Services), containing the Administration on Aging, the Social Security Administration, and many other bureaus; the Department of Housing and Urban Development; and the Department of Transportation. In addition to the thousands of divisions in these departments, there are some three thousand other advisory committees, boards, commissions, council, conferences, panels, task forces, and the like. A third group in the bureaucracy is the independent agencies. One such agency important to the elderly is the Federal Trade Commission.

The bureaucracies, or administrative agencies, are a major source of law—administrative law. Administrative law is of two types: First, agencies write "laws" of their own, called regulations. The authority of the agencies to pass regulations is found in the statutes creating the agencies. Regulations must always be viewed in the context of statutes—the sole function of the regulations must be to implement the statutes. There is another kind of law written by agencies in addition to regulations. These laws are often called administrative decisions. For example, if a dispute arises in the Social Security Administration about whether an individual is entitled to certain benefits, the agency has a procedure to resolve the controversy by holding a hearing and by writing a decision. Very often, the controversy involves interpretation of a statute as applied to a particular situation. Of course, the agency does not have final say on what the legislative intent of a statute is. If a citizen is dissatisfied with the interpretation given by the agency, the decision can usually be appealed to a court, which will make the definitive interpretation.

The Judicial Branch

Structure

Laws are merely statements of intention. Some agency must interpret them and apply them to specific problems. This is done by the courts.

The court system in the U.S. is like a pyramid. At the apex stands the U.S. Supreme Court, created by the Constitution. The Supreme Court consists of a chief justice and eight associate justices, nominated by the president and confirmed by the Senate. The bulk of the Supreme Court's work is appellate—reviewing decisions that come up on appeal from lower federal courts and from state courts. An example of a recent Supreme Court case affecting the elderly is *Massachusetts Board of Retirement* v. *Murgia*, 427 U.S. 302 (1976), which upheld a mandatory retirmenet age of 50 years for state police. Another is *Califano* v. *Goldfarb*, 45 U.S.L.W. 4237 (2 March 1977), in which the Supreme Court said that widowers should be able to get survivor's benefits from Social Security in the same way that widows get them.

Below the Supreme Court are the eleven U.S. courts of appeal, hearing appeals from the ninety-four U.S. district courts. The district courts are where most trials originate. Each state has at least one, and some have as many as four. The total workload for the over 400 judges is approaching 300,000 cases a year.

Each state has its own hierarchical system of courts, which often differ significantly from one another in structure, terminology, and distribution of powers. The base usually consists of a system of justices of the peace and trial courts (sometimes called county courts), then a more or less elaborate appellate system, culminating in a state supreme court.

Source of Law

On what do the courts rely to make their decisions? A study of the three branches of government and of the Constitution reveals the following sources of law. Judicial opinions are based in constitutional law, statutory law, administrative law—and common law. Common law is the set of laws that existed before statutory law, often deriving originally from decisions made in British courts long before the United States existed. It had its beginnings a thousand years ago in the creation of a legal system by the early nobles and kings. It is based on the idea of decision grounded in community norms and history. Judges may rule on the basis of these communal patterns as well as specific statutes or rules.

The judicial branch follows a doctrine known as *stare decisis*, which means that judges take into account past decisions of the court or of a higher court. This following of precedent assures uniformity in the law as it is applied to different people at different times. But the judge is also free to take account of historical changes in society, to find another precedent, or to interpret a statute—thus keeping the law a living thing.

Appendix B: Selected Organizations in Relation to the Aging

National Organizations

American Aging Association, University of Nebraska Medical Center, Omaha, Nebraska. Made up of scientists, it seeks to promote research in aging.

American Association of Homes for the Aging, 529 14th St., N.W., Washington, D.C., 20004. Represents the nonprofit homes for the aging—religious, municipal, trust, fraternal. AAHA includes voluntary nonprofit and governmental homes for the aging and other interested individuals and organizations; exists to provide unified means of identifying and solving problems of mutual concern so as to protect and advance the interests of the residents served; participates in a liaison with government in developing plans for basic curricula for administrators of homes; conducts institutes and workshops on current concerns such as accreditation, financing, and the meaning of institutional life and planning for the residents of the future. AAHA has several different publications and sponsors an annual convention.

American Association of Retired Persons, 1909 K Street, N.W., Washington, D.C., 20006. For age 55 or older, retired to still employed. AARP and National Retired Teachers Association have a membership of 2.7 million persons 55 years of age or older, whether or not retired. Their aim is to improve every aspect of living for older people. This organization has a library and several publications including *NRTA Journal* and *Dynamic Maturity*.

American Geriatrics Society, 10 Columbus Circle, New York, N.Y., 10010. Made up of physicians; has an annual meeting.

American Nursing Home Association (American Health Care Association), 1025 Connecticut Avenue, N.W., Washington, D.C., 20036. Represents the commercial nursing-home industry. A federation of state associations of nursing homes, this group includes profit and nonprofit homes. Prepares an annual compilation of nursing-home and bed totals and welfare payments by state. In addition to a 2,000-volume library, the association has several publications.

American Occupational Therapy Association, 251 Park Avenue South, New York, N.Y., 10010.

American Physical Therapy Association, 1740 Broadway, New York, N.Y., 10019.

227

American Public Welfare Association, 1313 East 60th Street, Chicago, Illinois, 60637. Has prepared teaching materials, anticipating the spread of gerontological training through universities and professional schools. Has a special committee to improve relations between welfare departments and aging.

Division of Adult Development and Aging: American Psychological Association, 1200 17th Street, N.W., Washington, D.C., 20036.

Forum for Professionals and Executives, Washington School of Psychiatry, 1610 New Hampshire Avenue, N.W., Washington, D.C., 20009. The interests of this group have ranged from contemplation to active examination of public issues, including those affecting the elderly.

Gerontological Society, Washington, D.C. 20036. This professional society has an annual meeting and an international meeting every three years. It is made up of four components: biological sciences, clinical medicine, psychological and social sciences, and social research, planning and practice. The Society is comprised of those interested in improving the well-being of older people by promoting scientific study of the aging process, publishing information about aging, and bringing together all groups interested in older people. Publishes the *Journal of Gerontology, The Gerontologist* and also what are referred to as *Selected Readings in Gerontology*, but these are not published regularly. In addition to being active in the publishing business, the Society sponsors an annual convention conference for all gerontologists and those interested in the field.

Gray Panthers, 6342 Greene Street, Philadelphia, Pennsylvania, 19144. Activistic group of old and young people who work together and fight against stereotyping.

Institute for Retired Professionals, The New School of Social Research, 60 West 12th Street, New York, N.Y. This pioneering school led the way in providing intellectual activities for retired professional people.

Institutes of Lifetime Learning. Educational Services of the National Retired Teachers Association and the American Association of Retired Persons.

International Federation on Aging, 1909 K Street, N.W., Washington, D.C., 20006. Confederation of aging organizations of various nations.

International Senior Citizens Association, Inc., 11753 Wilshire Boulevard, Los Angeles, California, 90025. Endeavors to reflect old people of many nations.

National Association of Retired Federal Employees, 1909 Q Street, N.W., Washington, D.C., 20009. Represents and lobbies for needs of retired civil servants.

National Association of Social Workers, 1425 H Street, N.W., Washington, D.C., 20005.

National Association of State Units on Aging. Address shifts as the presidency of the Association changes. The Association provides information resources on state policies on aging. Represents and lobbies for state agencies at the federal level.

National Caucus on the Black Aged, 1725 DeSales Street, N.W., Washington, D.C., 20036. Advocates improving quality of life of the black aged.

National Center on Black Aged, 1725 DeSales Street, N.W., Washington, D.C., 20036. Provides comprehensive program of coordination, information, and consultative services to meet needs of aged blacks.

National Council on the Aging, 1828 L Street, N.W., Suite 504, Washington, D.C., 20036. Research and services regarding the elderly. This is a voluntary agency that provides leadership services for organizations and individuals concerned with aid to the aging. It is nongovernmental, nonprofit, and tax exempt. It was organized in 1950 at the request of community leaders, civic groups, government agencies, and others who felt the need for professional advice and information in their field. NCOA sponsors the National Institute of Senior Centers (newsletter and bibliography available) and the National Institute on Industrial Gerontology, which publishes the journal *Industrial Gerontologist.* A catalog describing these and other publications is available from the National Council.

National Council of Health Care Services, 407 N Street, S.W., Washington, D.C. Represents commercial nursing-home chains.

National Council for Homemaker Services, 1790 Broadway, New York, N.Y., 10019.

National Council of Senior Citizens, 1911 K Street, N.W., Room 202, Washington, D.C., 20005. Represents and lobbies for needs of the elderly. Membership of any age. An organization of 3,000 autonomous senior citizens clubs, associations, councils, and other groups with a combined membership of over 3 million persons. It is an educational and action group that supports: medicare; increased social security; improved recreational, educational, and health programs; increased voluntary service programs; reduced costs on drugs; better housing; and other programs to aid senior citizens. Sponsors mass rallies, educational workshops, leadership training institutes; provides speakers on medicare or other problems concerning senior citizens; helps organize and develop programs for local and state groups. Encourages participation in social and political action activities; does not endorse candidates for political office but works on behalf of issues. Distributes films, news materials, special reports, and other materials. Maintains a library of books and collection of materials on medicare and other programs.

National Federation of Licensed Practical Nurses, 250 W. 57th Street, New York, N.Y. Educational foundation.

National Retired Teachers Association, 1909 K Street, N.W., Washington, D.C., 20006. Members once active in an educational system, public or private.

National Tenants Organization, Inc., Suite 548, 425 13th Street, N.W., Washington, D.C., 20004. Represents old people, among others, in public housing.

Oliver Wendell Holmes Association, 381 Park Avenue South, New York, N.Y., 10016. This group is interested in the expansion of the intellectual horizons of older people.

Retired Professional Action Group, Suite 711, 200 P Street, N.W., Washington, D.C. This action group was organized through Ralph Nader. Its efforts include investigative reports and class-action cases.

Urban Elderly Coalition, c/o Office of Aging of New York City, 250 Broadway, New York, N.Y. Effort of municipal authorities to obtain funds for the urban elderly poor.

Federal Agencies

Administration on Aging, 330 Independence Avenue, Washington, D.C., 20201. AOA is defined as administering grant programs to states designed to stimulate the development of public and private services and opportunities for older people at state and local levels. It directs a program to provide for the training of manpower in the field of aging. The Administration serves as a clearing house for information related to the aging and the aged; maintains relationships with and provides guidance, consultation, and technical program assistance to federal, state, and local organizations that serve or have an impact on the aging and the aged; analyzes and comments on legislative proposals from other services affecting older people; and evaluates progress and promotes improvement in national programs to meet the needs of older people.

Bureau of Labor Statistics, Washington, D.C., 20212. This office is a very good source for figures and statistics on income, employment, and budgets relating to the older population.

Bureau of Labor Statistics, Washington, D.C., 20212. This office is a very good source for figures and statistics on income, employment, and budgets relating to the older population.

Department of Commerce, Social and Economics Statistics Administration, U.S. Bureau of the Census, Suitland, Maryland, 20233. This office is responsible for the publication of a series of reports called *Current Population Reports*, which contain all kinds of data and would be most useful to anyone wanting to describe the older population. Statistics for

Check with the Bureau of Census for a listing of the series to see which ones you might be interested in acquiring.

National Institute on Aging of the U.S. Department of Health, Education and Welfare, Public Health Service, National Institutes of Health, Bethseda, Maryland, 20014. This institute was established in 1974 to conduct and support biomedical, social, and behavioral research and training related to the aging process as well as diseases and other special problems and needs of the aged.

Select House Committee on the Aging, House of Representatives, Washington, D.C., 20510.

Senate Special Committee on Aging, Senate Office Building, Washington, D.C., 20510. This Committe publishes a comprehensive list of the hearings, studies, and working papers they have conducted and sponsored in the past year. Of particuilar importance is *Developments in Aging* issued at the end of each year and containing the best all-around description of what has transpired in the field of aging during the previous year. This information is available to individuals free of charge.

Social Security Administration, Office of Research and Statistics. This office publishes valuable reports regarding the trends of the aging population of the United States. It publishes the *Social Security Bulletin*, which includes a comprehensive annual report on the social security program.

**Appendix C:
Federal Programs
Benefiting the Aged
(1978)**

Federal Agencies Administering Selected Programs for the Aging

Executive Departments — Agriculture (Farmers Home Administration; Food and Nutrition Service); Health and Human Services (Health Services Administration; Social Security Administration; Office of Education; Administration for Public Services; Administration on Aging; Health Care Financing Administration; National Institute of Mental Health; National Institute on Aging); Housing and Urban Development (Office of Insured and Direct Loan Programs; Assisted Housing; Community Planning and Development); Labor (Employment Standards Administration; Employment and Training Administration); Transportation (Urban Mass Transportation Administration; Federal Highway Administration); TREASURY (Office of Revenue Sharing); Action; Community Services Administration; Legal Services Corporation

Independent Agencies — Railroad Retirement Board; Small Business Administration; U.S. Civil Service Commission; Veterans Administration

Program	Health Services Admin.	Health Care Financing Admin.	Office of Insured & Direct Loan Programs	Employment Standards Admin.	Employment & Training Admin.	Action	Community Services Admin.	Legal Services Corp.	Small Business Admin.	U.S. Civil Service Commission	Veterans Administration
Employment											
Age Discrimination in Employment				•						•	
Employment Programs for Special Groups					•						
Foster Grandparent Program						•					
Older Americans Community Service Employment Program					•						
Retired-Senior Volunteer Program (RSVP)						•					
Service Corps of Retired Executives (SCORE)								•			
Volunteers in Service to America (VISTA)						•					
Health Care											
Health Resources Development Construction and Modernization of Facilities (Hill-Burton Prog)	•										
Construction of Nursing Homes and Intermediate Care Facilities			•								
Grants to States for Medical Assistance Programs (Medicaid)		•									
Program of Health Insurance for the Aged and Disabled (Medicare)		•									
Veterans Domiciliary Care Program											•
Veterans Nursing-Home Care Program											•

Veterans Nursing-Home Care Program

Community Mental Health Centers

Housing

Housing for the Elderly (Sec. 202 of Federal Housing Act of 1968)

Low- and Moderate-Income Housing (Sec. 8 of Federal Housing Act of 1970)

Mortgage Insurance on Rental Housing for the Elderly (Sec. 231 of Federal Housing Act of 1974)

Rural Rental Housing Loans

Community Development

Rental and Cooperative Housing for Lower and Moderate-Income Families (Sec. 236 of Federal Housing Act of 1974)

Congregate Housing

Income Maintenance

Civil Service Retirement

Old-Age, Survivors Insurance Programs (Social Security)

Railroad Retirement Program

Supplemental Security Income Program

Veterans Pension Program

Food Stamp Program

Social Service Programs

Education Programs for Non-English-Speaking Elderly

Legal Services Corporation

Model Projects

Multipurpose Senior Centers

Nutrition Program for the Elderly

Older-Reader Services

Revenue Sharing

Column groupings (department headers):

Executive Departments

- Agriculture: Farmers Home Administration; Food and Nutrition Service; Health Services Administration; Social Security Administration; Office of Education
- Health and Human Services: Administration for Public Services; Administration on Aging; Health Care Financing Administration; National Institute of Mental Health; National Institute on Aging; Office of Insured and Direct Loan Programs; Office of Housing and Assisted Housing
- Housing and Urban Development: Community Planning and Development; Employment Standards Administration; Employment and Training Administration
- Labor: Urban Mass Transportation Administration; Federal Highway Administration
- Transportation: TREASURY — Office of Revenue Sharing; Action
- Independent Agencies: Community Services Corporation; Legal Services Administration; Railroad Retirement Board; Small Business Administration; U.S. Civil Service Commission; Veterans Administration

Row labels (programs):

- Senior Opportunities and Services
- Social Services for Low-Income Persons and Public Assistance Recipients (Title XX)
- State and Community Programs (Title III)

Training and Research Programs
- Multidisciplinary Centers of Gerontology
- Nursing Home Care, Training, and Research Programs
- Personnel Training
- Research and Demonstration Program
- Research on Aging Process and Health Problems
- Research on Problems of the Elderly

Transportation
- Reduced Fares
- Capital Assistance Grants for Public Agencies
- Capital Assistance Grants for Private Nonprofit Groups
- Rural Highway Public Transportation Demonstration Project

Source: Printed for the use of the Select Committee on Aging (Washington, D.C.: U.S. Government Printing Office, 1977).

**Appendix D: Senate
and House Committees
and Subcommittees
with Jurisdiction over
Areas Related to the
Elderly**

Senate Committees and Subcommittees

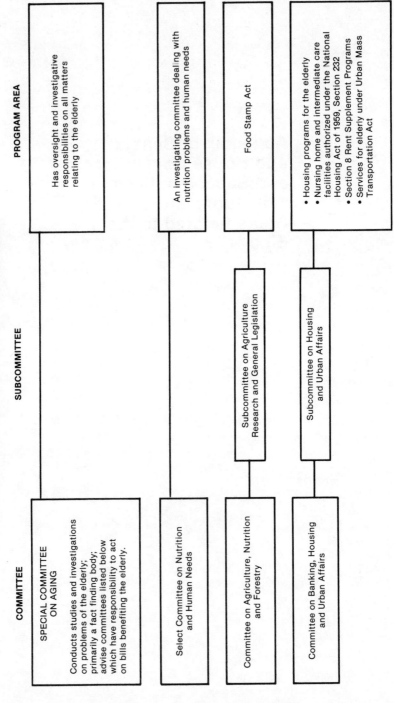

COMMITTEE	SUBCOMMITTEE	PROGRAM AREA
SPECIAL COMMITTEE ON AGING Conducts studies and investigations on problems of the elderly; primarily a fact finding body; advise committees listed below which have responsibility to act on bills benefiting the elderly.		Has oversight and investigative responsibilities on all matters relating to the elderly
Select Committee on Nutrition and Human Needs		An investigating committee dealing with nutrition problems and human needs
Committee on Agriculture, Nutrition and Forestry	Subcommittee on Agriculture Research and General Legislation	Food Stamp Act
Committee on Banking, Housing and Urban Affairs	Subcommittee on Housing and Urban Affairs	• Housing programs for the elderly • Nursing home and intermediate care facilities authorized under the National Housing Act of 1959, Section 232 • Section 8 Rent Supplement Programs • Services for elderly under Urban Mass Transportation Act

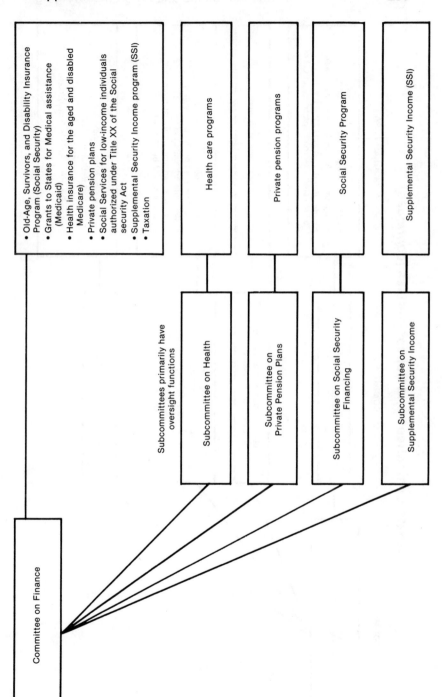

Committee on Finance

- Old-Age, Survivors, and Disability Insurance Program (Social Security)
- Grants to States for Medical assistance (Medicaid)
- Health insurance for the aged and disabled (Medicare)
- Private pension plans
- Social Services for low-income individuals authorized under Title XX of the Social security Act
- Supplemental Security Income program (SSI)
- Taxation

Health care programs

Private pension programs

Social Security Program

Supplemental Security Income (SSI)

Subcommittees primarily have oversight functions

Subcommittee on Health

Subcommittee on Private Pension Plans

Subcommittee on Social Security Financing

Subcommittee on Supplemental Security Income

Senate Committees and Subcommittees *(continued)*

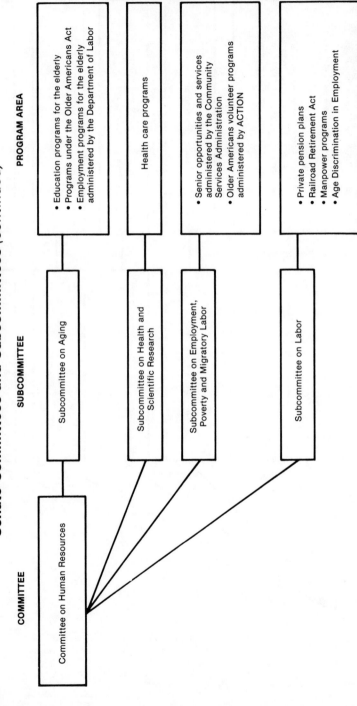

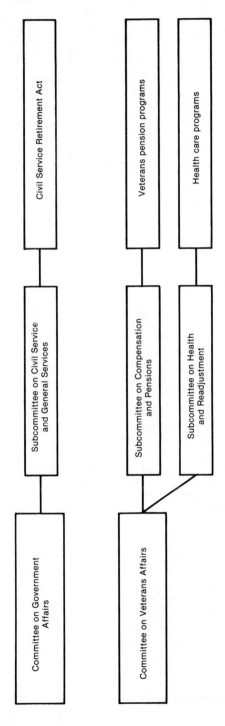

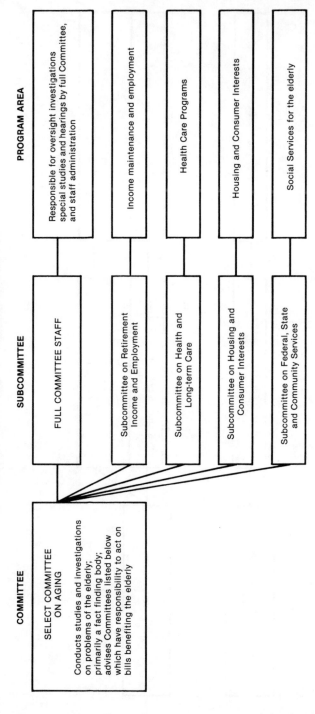

House Committees and Subcommittees

COMMITTEE

SELECT COMMITTEE ON AGING

Conducts studies and investigations on problems of the elderly; primarily a fact finding body; advises Committees listed below which have responsibility to act on bills benefitting the elderly

SUBCOMMITTEE

FULL COMMITTEE STAFF

Subcommittee on Retirement Income and Employment

Subcommittee on Health and Long-term Care

Subcommittee on Housing and Consumer Interests

Subcommittee on Federal, State and Community Services

PROGRAM AREA

Responsible for oversight investigations special studies and hearings by full Committee, and staff administration

Income maintenance and employment

Health Care Programs

Housing and Consumer Interests

Social Services for the elderly

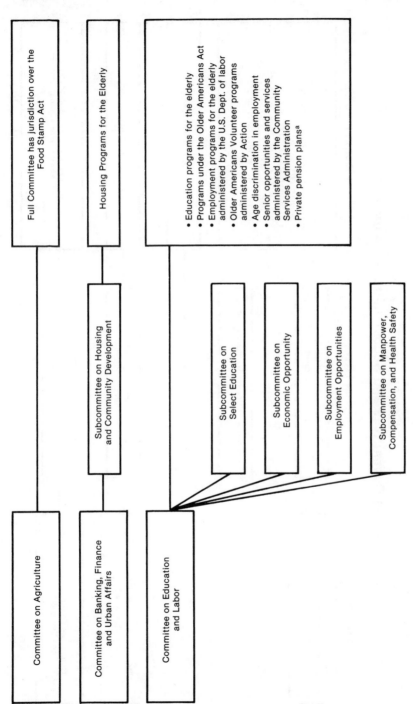

House Committees and Subcommittees *(continued)*

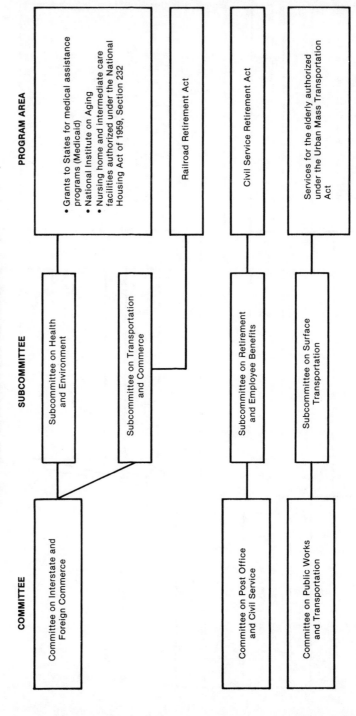

COMMITTEE

Committee on Interstate and Foreign Commerce

Committee on Post Office and Civil Service

Committee on Public Works and Transportation

SUBCOMMITTEE

Subcommittee on Health and Environment

Subcommittee on Transportation and Commerce

Subcommittee on Retirement and Employee Benefits

Subcommittee on Surface Transportation

PROGRAM AREA

• Grants to States for medical assistance programs (Medicaid)
• National Institute on Aging
• Nursing home and intermediate care facilities authorized under the National Housing Act of 1959, Section 232

Railroad Retirement Act

Civil Service Retirement Act

Services for the elderly authorized under the Urban Mass Transportation Act

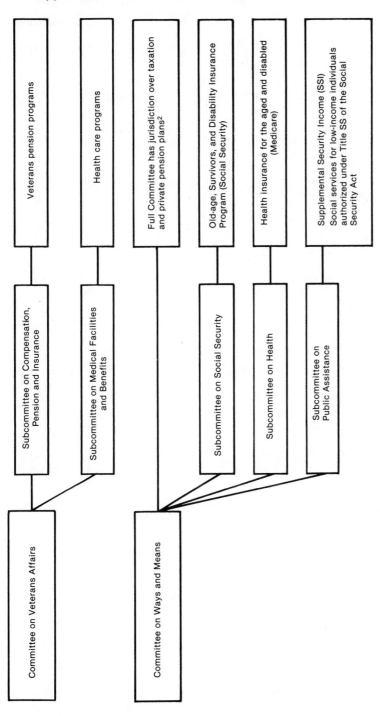

Note: Jurisdiction over subject matters listed not permanently assigned to specific subcommittees.

[a]Bills on pension plans are referred either to Committee on Education and Labor or Committee on Ways and Means, depending upon content of bill.

Appendix E:
Outline for a
Descriptive Analysis
of Social Welfare
Programs

1. Goals of Program: What social need or social problem does program address?
2. Nature of Program: How does it address this need or problem? Is it residual, institutional, or developmental in orientation? Is it curative, preventive, or enhancement oriented?
3. Scope of Program: What is the extent and size of the program? Who is the target population? How many people or population groups are affected by the program? What are the eligibility requirements? Who is excluded?
4. Auspices: Under whose auspices does it operate (government, voluntary, sectarian, or nonsectarian; any combination)? Which agencies operate this program?
5. Functions, Coverage, and Operations: How does the program function? How does it actually operate?
6. Beneficiaries: Who are the actual beneficiaries of the program?
7. Benefits: What are the services and/or benefits? To what extent are the services/benefits adequate? To what extent are they equitable?
8. Delivery: How are the benefits or services delivered to the people or population groups? What are the major obstacles to the delivery of benefits or services to making them available, accessible and acceptable?
9. Organization, Management, and Personnel: What organizational arrangements, structures and mechanisms exist to operate the programs? Who administers and delivers these programs/services? What are the qualifications and preparations for those who deliver and administer the services? How adequate are these?
10. Financing: What sources of funding are used? How are these sources used to finance the program (federal, state, local, private)? What is the flow of these funding sources (from federal to state to municipality) by grants or contracts, by donations, gifts or contributions? How do funding sources and funding flow affect program directions and service delivery?
11. Evaluation: What evaluation and monitoring mechanisms are used to assess program/service management, organization and impact? Who is involved in evaluation and monitoring procedures? How are results of evaluations utilized?

Bibliography

Atchley, Robert. *The Social Forces in Later Life*. 3d ed. Belmont, Calif: Wadsworth Publishing, 1979.

Baum, Martha and Rainer C. Baum. *Growing Old: A Societal Perspective*. Englewood Cliffs, N.J.: Prentice-Hall, 1980.

Beattie, Walter M., Jr. "Aging and the Social Services," in R. Binstock and E. Shanas, eds., Handbook of *Aging and the Social Sciences*. New York: Van Nostrand, Reinhold, 1978, chap. 24.

Bellack, L. and H. Barten, (eds.) *Progress in Community Mental Health*. New York: Grune and Stratton, 1969.

Bengtson, Vern. *The Social Psychology of Aging*. New York: Bobbs-Merrill, 1973.

Binstock, Robert. "Interest-group Liberalism and the Politics of Aging," *The Gerontologist* 12 (Autumn 1972):265-280.

———— . "Aging and the Future of American Politics," *The Annals of the American Academy of Political Science* 415 (1974):199-212.

Binstock, Robert and R. Hudson. "Political Systems and Aging," in R.H. Binstock and E. Shanas, eds., *Handbook of Aging and the Social Sciences*. New York: Van Nostrand, Reinhold, 1976.

Binstock, Robert H. and Martin A. Levin. "The Political Dilemma of Intervention Policies," in Robert H. Binstock and Ethel Shanas, eds., *Handbook of Aging and the Social Sciences*. New York: Van Nostrand, Reinhold, 1976, pp. 511-535.

Binstock, Robert H. and Ethel Shanas, eds. *Handbook of Aging and the Social Sciences*. New York: Van Nostrand, Reinhold, 1976.

Birren, James E. and R. Bruce Sloane (eds.) *Handbook of Mental Health and Aging*. Englewood N.J.: Prentice-Hall, 1980.

Blenkner, Margaret. "Social Work and Family Relationships in Later Years with Some Thoughts on Filial Maturity," in Ethel Shanas and Gordon F. Streib, eds., *Social Structure and the Family: Generational Relations*. Englewood Cliffs, N.J.: Prentice-Hall, 1965.

Borges, M. and L. Dutton. "Attitudes toward Aging: Increasing Optimism Found with Age," *Gerontologist* 16 (1976): 236-242.

Bracht, Neil. *Social Work in Health Care: A Guide to Professional Practice*. New York: Hayworth Press, 1978.

Brody, Elaine M. "The Aging Family," *The Gerontologist* 6 (1966): pp. 201-206.

———— . *A Social Work Guide for Long-term Care Facilities*. Rockville, Md.: National Institute of Mental Health, 1974.

———— . "Aging," *Encyclopedia of Social Work*. Washington, D.C.: National Association of Social Workers, 1977.

Brody, Elaine M. and Stanley J. Brody. "Decade of Decision for the Elder-
    ly," *Social Work*, (September 1974): Vol. 19 No. 5, 544-554.
Brody, Stanley J. *A Preventive Mental Health Program for the Elderly*.
    Background Issues Paper prepared for the Committee on Mental
    Health and Illness of the Elderly, 1977.
_____ . "Comprehensive Health Care for the Elderly: An Analysis,"
    Gerontologist 13 (1973):412-418.
Burnside, Irene M. *Working with the Elderly: Group Processes and Tech-
    niques*. Belmont, Calif.: Duxbury Press, 1978.
Butler, Robert. *Why Survive? Being Old in America*. New York: Harper
    and Row, 1975.
Butler, Robert and Lewis Myrna. *Aging and Mental Health*. 2d ed. St.
    Louis: C.V. Mosby, 1977.
Cantor, Marjorie H. *The Elderly in the Inner City*. New York: New York
    City Office for the Aging, 1973.
Cantor, Marjorie H. and M.J. Mayer. "Factors in Differential Utilization
    of Urban Elderly," *Journal of Gerontological Social Work* 1,
    (1978):49-50, 59.
Carp, Frances M. "Impact of Improved Housing on Morale and Life Satis-
    faction," *Gerontologist* 15 (1975):511-515.
Carp, Frances M. "The Concept and Role of Congregate Housing for
    Older People," *Congregate Housing for Older People*. Prepared for
    the Department of Health, Education and Welfare. Washington, D.C.:
    International Center for Social Gerontology, 1977.
Cohen, Gene D. "Mental Health and the Elderly," Unpublished issues
    paper, NIMH. Rockville, Md.: Center for Studies of the Mental Health
    of the Aging, 1977.
Comfort, Alex. *A Good Age*. New York: Crown Publishers, 1976.
Commerce Clearing House, Inc. *1974 Social Security and Medicare Ex-
    plained*, 1974.
Congressional Budget Office. *Long-Term Care for the Elderly and Dis-
    abled*. Washington, D.C., February 1977.
_____ . *Long-Term Care: Actuarial Cost Estimates*. Washington,
    D.C., August 1977.
Cumming, Elaine and Henry William. *Growing Old—The Process of Dis-
    engagement*. New York: Basic Books, 1961.
Curtin, Sharon R. *Nobody Ever Died of Old Age*. Boston: Little,
    Brown, 1972.
de Beauvoir, Simone. *The Coming of Age*. New York: Warner Paperback
    Library, 1970.
DeCordova Museum School of Art. *Report*. Lincoln, Massachusetts,
    1979.
Estes, Carroll L. *The Aging Enterprise*. San Francisco: Jossey-Bass, 1979.

Etzioni, Amitai. "Old People and Public Policy," *Social Policy* Vol. 7 No. 3 (November/December 1976):21-29.

Federal Council on the Aging. *The Impact of the Tax Structure on the Elderly*. Washington, D.C., December 1975.

Fisher, David H. "The Politics of Aging in America, a Short History," *The Journal of the Institute of Socio-Economic Studies* 4 (Summer 1979):51-66.

Frankfather, Dwight. *The Aged in the Community*. New York: Praeger, 1977.

Freeman, Howard E. and Clarence C. Sherwood. *Social Research and Social Policy*. Englewood Cliffs, N.J.: Prentice-Hall, 1970.

Gelwicks, Louis E. and Robert J. Newcomer. *Planning Housing Environments for the Elderly*. Washington, D.C.: National Council on the Aging, 1974.

General Accounting Office. *Home Health—The Need for a National Policy to Provide for the Elderly*. Washington, D.C., 30 December 1977.

_____ . *Returning the Mentally Disabled to the Community: Government Needs to Do More*. Washington, D.C., January 1977.

Gilbert, Neil and Harry Specht. *Dimensions of Social Welfare Policy*. Englewood, N.J.: Prentice-Hall, 1974.

Golant, Stephen M., Ph.D., and Rosemary McCaslin, M.A. "A Functional Classification of Services for Older People," *Journal of Gerontological Social Work*, 1 (Spring 1979):187-202.

Gurian, Bennett. *Current and Anticipated Need for Mental Services and Service Facilities to Meet the Mental Health Care Needs of the Elderly*. Background issue paper prepared for the Committee on Mental Health and Illness of the Elderly, under contract to the Gerontological Society, 1977.

Gutman, G. and C. Herbert. "Mortality Rates among Relocated Extended Care Patients," *Journal of Gerontology* 31 (1976):352-357.

Hall, Gertrude H. and Geneva Mathiasen. *Guide to Development of Protective Services for Older People*. Springfield, Ill.: Charles C. Thomas, Bannerstone House, 1973.

Harris, Charles S. *Fact Book on Aging: A Profile on America's Older Population*. Washington, D.C.: National Council on the Aging, February 1978.

Harris, Diana and William E. Cole. *Sociology of Aging*. Boston: Houghton Mifflin, 1980.

Harris, Samuel E., et al. *Alternatives to Institutionalization of the Elderly—The State of the Art*. Washington, D.C.: Sam Harris Associates, January 1976.

Hudson, Robert. "The Graying of the Federal Budget and Its Consequences for Old Age Policy," *The Gerontologist* 18 (October 1978):428-440.

Human Resources Corporation. *Policy Issues Concerning the Minority Elderly*. Contracted by the Federal Council on the Aging. Washington, D.C., 1978.

Kahana, Eva and Rodney Coe. "Alternatives in Long Term Care," in Sylvia Sherwood, ed., *Long Term Care, A Guide for Researchers and Planners*. Chapter 11, pp. 511-572. New York: Spectrum Publishers, 1975.

Kahn, Alfred J. and Sheila B. Kamerman. *Not for the Poor Alone: European Social Services*. Philadelphia: Temple University Press, 1975.

Kahn, Robert. "The Mental Health System and the Future Aged," *Social Problems of the Aging*. in M. Seltzer, S. Corbett, R. Atchley, eds., Belmont, Calif.: Wadsworth Publishing, 1978.

Kalish, R.A., ed. "Aging and Ethnicity," *The Later Years*. Monterey, Calif.: Brooks/Cole Publishing, 1977.

Kamerman, Sheila B. "Community Services for the Aged: The View from Eight Countries," *The Gerontologist* 16 (1976):529-537.

Kamerman, Sheila and Alfred Kahn. *Social Services in the United States*. Philadelphia: Temple University Press, 1976.

Kane, Robert L. and Rosalie A. Kane. "Care of the Aged: Old Problems in Need of New Solutions," *Science* 200 (May 1978):pp. 910-919.

Kaplan, Max. *Leisure: Lifestyle and Lifespan*. Philadelphia: W.B. Saunders, 1979.

Kart, Cary S. and Barbara Manard, eds. *Aging in America: Readings in Social Gerontology*. Ft. Washington, N.J.: Alfred Publishing, 1976.

Kastenbaum, Robert. "The Reluctant Therapist," *New Thoughts on Old Age*. New York: Springer, 1964.

Kerschner, Paul A., ed. *Advocacy and Age*. Los Angeles: University of Southern California Press, 1976.

Kluckohn, Florence. "Dominant and Variant Value Orientations," *Personality in Nature, Society, and Culture*. New York: Alfred A. Knopf, 1953.

Kreps, Juanita. "The Economy and the Aged," in Robert H. Binstock and Ethel Shanas, eds., *Handbook of Aging and The Social Sciences*. New York: Van Nostrand, Reinhold, 1976.

———. "Intergenerational Transfers and the Bureaucracy," in Ethel Shanas and Marvin B. Sussman, eds., *Family, Bureaucracy and the Elderly*. Durham, N.C.: Duke University Press, 1977.

Krueger, Gladys. "Financing of Mental Health Care of the Aged.", Paper prepared under NIMH contract for the Committee on Mental Health and Illness of the Elderly, 1977.

Kubey, Robert W. "Television and Aging: Past, Present and Future," *The Gerontologist* 20 (February 1980): 16-35.

Kuhn, Margaret E. "Open Letter," *The Gerontologist* (1978): 422-424.

Lack, Sylvia. "Referral: Hospice," in R. Kalish, ed., *The Later Years: Social Applications of Gerontology*. Monterey, Calif.: Brooks Cole, Publishing, 1977.

Lakoff, Sanford. "The Future of Social Intervention," in R. Binstock and E. Shanas, eds., *Aging and Social Sciences*. New York: Van Nostrand, Reinhold, 1976.

Law and Aging Manual, Washington D.C.: National Council of Senior Citizens, 1976.

Legislative Council for Older Americans, "Statement," Boston, Massachusetts.

Lifeline, An Emergency Alarm System. Report to the Health Care Finance Administration. Boston: Hebrew Rehabilitation Center for the Aged, 1980.

Little, Virginia. "Open Care for the Aging: Alternate Approaches," *Aging*. Washington, D.C.: U.S. Department of Health, Education and Welfare, Administration on Aging, November-December 1979.

Lowy, Louis. "Models for Organization of Services to the Aging," *Aging and Human Development* 1 (1970): pp. 21-36.

_____. "A Social Work Practice Perspective in Relation to Theoretical Models and Research in Gerontology," in Donald P. Kent, Robert Kastenbaum, and Sylvia Sherwood, eds., *Research Planning and Action for the Elderly*. New York: Behavioral Publications, 1972.

_____. "The Senior Center, a Community Facility," *Perspective*, Vol. 3, No. 2 (March/April 1974) pp. 5-9.

Lowy, Louis. "Social Welfare and the Aging," in M. Spencer and J. Dorr eds., *Understanding Aging*. New York: Appleton-Century-Crofts, 1975.

_____. "Adult Children and Their Parents: Dependency or Dependability," *Long Term Care and Health Services Administration Quarterly*, Fall 1977; pp. 243-248.

_____. *Social Work with the Aging: The Challenge and the Promise of the Later Years*. New York: Harper and Row, 1979.

Lowy, Louis and Margot Helphand. "Matching Community Resources and Patient Needs," in Sylvia Sherwood, ed., *Long-Term Care: A Handbook for Researchers, Planners and Providers*. New York: Spectrum Publications, 1975.

McCamman, Dorothy. "The Role of Private Pensions in Providing Retirement Income in the United States." in *Income in Retirement* 1975 (New York: Institute of Life Insurance) pp. 100-120.

Maddox, George L. "Self Assessment of Health Status: A Longitudinal Study of Selected Elderly Subjects," *Journal of Chronic Diseases* 17 (1964): 449-460.

Maslow, Abraham H. *Motivation and Personality*. New York: Harper and Row, 1954.

Materials on the Supplemental Security Income Program. National Senior Citizens Law Center. Los Angeles, Calif., December 1974.

Mendelson, Mary. *Tender Loving Greed.* New York: Vintage Books, Random House, 1974.

Mental Health and the Elderly. Reports of the President's Commission on Mental Health: Task panels on the Elderly and the Secretary's Committee on the Mental Health and Illness of the Elderly. Washington, D.C.: U.S. Department of Health, Education and Welfare, Federal Council on Aging, 1978.

Morris, Robert. "Aging and the Field of Social Work," in Matilda Riley, Anne Foner, Mary E. Moore, Beth Hess, and Barbara K. Roth, eds., *Aging and Society,* vol. 2. New York: Russell Sage Foundation, 1969.

Morris, Robert. *Social Policy of the American Welfare State.* New York: Harper and Row, 1979.

Morris, Robert and Delwin Anderson. "Personal Care Services: An Identity for Social Work," *Social Service Review.* 1975.

Murray, Roger F. "Economic Aspects of Pensions: A Summary Report," *U.S. Joint Economic Committee, Old Age Income Assurance,* part V. Washington D.C.: U.S. Government Printing Office, 1967.

Myers, Robert J. "Government and Pensions," *Private Pensions and the Public Interest.* Washington, D.C.: American Enterprise Institute for the Public Policy Research, 1970.

Nagi, Saad Z. *An Epidemiology of Disability among Adults in the United States.* Columbus, Ohio: Ohio State University, 1975.

Nagi, Saad Z. and Berenice King. *Aging and the Organization of Services.* Columbus, Ohio: Mershon Center, Ohio State University, 1976.

National Association of Social Workers. *News.* February 1980.

National Council on Aging. *Directory of Senior Centers and Clubs.* Washington, D.C., 1975.

_____ . *Fact Book on Aging.* Washington, D.C., 1976.

_____ . *The Myth and Reality of Aging in America.* Washington, D.C., 1976.

Neugarten, Bernice L. and Robert I. Havighurst, eds. *Social Policy, Social Ethics and the Aging Society.* Washington, D.C.: U.S. Government Printing Office, 1976.

No Longer Young: The Older Woman in America. Work Group reports from the 26th Conference on Aging, Institute of Gerontology, University of Michigan, Wayne State University, 1975.

Older American Reports, February 1980. Washington, D.C.: Capitol Publications.

Older Americans Act: A Summary. Staff study, Select Committee on Aging, U.S. House of Representatives, August 1978.

Older Americans Act of 1965, As Amended. P. L. 95-178 Administration on Aging, July 1979. DHEW Publication, Washington, D.C.

Osterbond, Carter C. "Income in Retirement: The Need and Society's Responsibility." Report on the 16th Annual Southern Conference on Gerontology, University of Florida, Institute of Gerontology. Gainsville: University of Florida Press, 1967.

Paillat, Paul. "Bureaucratization of Old Age: Determinants of the Process, Possible Safeguards and Reorientation," in Ethel Shanas and Marvin B. Sussman, eds., *Family, Bureaucracy and the Elderly*. Durham, N.C.: Duke University Press, 1977.

Palmore, Erdman and Kenneth Manton. "Ageism Compared to Racism and Sexism," in Seltzer, Corbett, and Atchley, eds., *Social Problems of the Aging*. Belmont, Calif.: Wadsworth Publishing, 1978.

Palmore, Erdman B. and Kenneth Manton. "Ageism Compared to Racism and Sexism," *Journal of Gerontology* 38 (1973): 353-369.

Parsons, Talcott. "The Professions and Social Structure," *Social Forces* 17 (1939): 457-467.

Pension Policy Commission Act. (PL 96-14).

Pfeiffer, Eric, M.D. *Alternatives to Institutional Care for Older Americans: Practice and Planning*. Durham, N.C.: Center for the Study of Aging and Human Development, 1973.

Powell, Lawton M. *Planning and Managing Housing for the Elderly*. New York: J. Wiley and Sons, 1975.

President's Task Force on Aging. *Report on Nutrition*. Washington, D.C., 1970.

Rawls, John. *Social Justice*. Cambridge, Mass.: Harvard University Press, 1971.

Rosencrantz, H. and I. McNevin. "A Factor Analysis of Attitudes Toward the Aged," *Gerontologist 9* (1971): 55-59.

Rosow, Irving. *Social Integration of the Aged*. New York: The Free Press, 1967.

——— . *Socialization to Old Age*. Berkeley and Los Angeles: University of California Press, 1974.

Schottland, Charles I. *The Social Security Program in the United States*. 1970.

Schulz, James H. *Pension Aspects of the Economics of Aging: Present and Future Roles of Private Pensions*. Committee Print, U.S. Senate Special Committee on Aging. Washington, D.C.: U.S. Governmental Printing Office, 1970.

——— . "The Economic Impact of an Aging Population," *Gerontologist* 13 (1973): 111-117.

——— . *The Economics of Aging*. 2d ed. Belmont, Calif.: Wadsworth Publishing Company, 1979.

Schulz, James H., Guy Carrin, Hans Krupp, Manfred Peschke, Eliot Sclar, J. Van Steenberge. *Providing Adequate Retirement Income-Pension Reform in the United Ststes and Abroad*. Hanover, N.H.: Brandeis University Press/New England Press, 1974.

Seltzer, Mildred, Sherry Corbett, Robert Atchley, eds., *Social Problems of Aging*. Belmont, Calif.: Wadsworth Publishing, 1978.

Senate Special Committee on Aging, *Future Directions in Social Security—Unresolved Issues: An Interim Staff Report*. Washington, D.C., 1975.

Shanas, Ethel and George L. Maddox. "Aging, Health and the Organization Health Resources," in R.H. Binstock and E. Shanas, eds., *Handbook of Aging and the Social Sciences*. New York: Van Nostrand, Reinhold, 1976.

Shanas, Ethel and Marvin B. Sussman. *Family, Bureaucracy, and the Elderly*. Durham, N.C.: Duke University Press, 1977.

Shanas, E., P. Townsend, D. Wedderburn, H. Friis, P. Milhøj, J. Stehouwer. *Old People in Three Industrial Societies*. New York: Atherton Press; London: Routledge & Kegan Paul, 1968.

Sherwood, Sylvia, ed. *Long-Term Care: A Handbook for Researchers, Planners and Providers*. New York: Spectrum Publications, 1975.

Social Security Act, (Title II), *U.S. Code*, starting at 42 USC 401. Social Security benefit regulations are contained in Part 404 of Title XX of the *Code of Federal Regulations*.

Social Security Act, Title 18, ("Medicare"), U.S. Code at 42 U.S.C., sec. 1395. The Medicare regulations, promulgated by the Social Security Administration, may be found in the *Code of Federal Regulations* at 20 C.F.R., sec. 404.

Social Security Act, Title 19, (Medicaid), Volume 42 U.S.C., sec. 1396. The federal regulations that apply to the state operation of medicaid are published in vol. 45 of the *Code of Federal Regulations*, secs. 246-250. The regulations governing the operation of medicaid within a particular state are issued by that state.

Social Security Administration. *Social Security Programs throughout the World*. Office of Research and Statistics Research Report No. 44. Washington, D.C.: U.S. Government Printing Office, 1973.

"Social-Cultural Contexts of Aging: Implications for Social Policy." Andrus Gerontology Center, University of Southern California, Los Angeles, California, 1976.

Special Committee on Aging, U.S. Senate. *Hearing on Effectiveness of Food Stamps for Older Americans*. Superintendent of Documents. Washington, D.C.: U.S. Government Printing Office, 19 April 1977.

Streib, Gordon and G.J. Schneider. *Retirement in American Society*. Ithaca, N.Y.: Cornell University Press, 1971.

Tobin, Sheldon. "Social and Health Services for the Future Aged," *The Gerontologist* 15 (1975): 32-37.

Tobin, Sheldon S., Stephen M. Davidson, and Ann Sack. *Effective Social Services for Older Americans*. Ann Arbor, Mich.: Institute of Gerontology, 1976.

Tobin, Sheldon S. and Morton St. Lieberman. *Last Home for the Aged.* San Francisco, Calif.: Jossey-Bass, 1976.

United Nations. *The Aging: Trends and Policies.* New York: United Nations Press, 1975.

U.S. Bureau of Census, *Current Population Reports.* Ser. P-20, no. 338 and earlier reports, ser. P-23, nos. 57, 59, ser. P-23, no. 800, and ser. P-80, nos. 118, 119. Washington, D.C., 1976.

_____ . *Current Population Reports.* Ser. P-25, nos. 519, 724, and 800. Washington, D.C., 1977.

_____ . "Characteristics of the Population below the Poverty Level: 1976," *Current Population Reports.* Ser. P-60, no. 115. Washington, D.C., July 1978.

U.S. Civil Rights Commission. *Age Discrimination Study.* Superintendent of Documents (Washington, D.C., 1977).

U.S. Congressional Budget. U.S. Governmental Document Publication. Washington, D.C.: U.S. Government Printing Office, 1977.

U.S. Department of Agriculture, Food and Nutrition Service. *The Food Stamp Program.* Washington, D.C.

U.S. Department of Health, Education and Welfare, Administration on Aging, *Let's End Isolation.* DHEW Publication (OHDS) 78-20129. Washington, D.C., 1973.

U.S. Department of Health, Education and Welfare, Health Resources Administration, National Center for Health Statistics. *Health United States — 1976-1977.* Washington, D.C., 1977.

U.S. Department of Health, Education and Welfare, Office of Human Development Services. *Facts about Older Americans*, DHEW Publication (OHDS) 79-20006. Washington, D.C., 1978.

U.S. Department of Health, Education, and Welfare, Social Security Administration. *Social Security Programs around the World.* Washington, D.C., 1973.

U.S. Department of Health, Education and Welfare, Federal Council on Aging. *Public Policy and the Frail Elderly.* DHEW Publication (OHDS) 79-20959. Washington D.C., 1978.

U.S. Department of Housing and Urban Development. *"How Well are We Housed? The Elderly.* Washington, D.C.: U.S. Government Printing Office, 1977.

U.S. General Accounting Office. *The Well-Being of Older People in Cleveland, Ohio.* Washington, D.C., April 1977.

U.S. House Select Committee on Aging, U.S. House of Representatives, *Economic Problems of Aging Women, Hearings before the Subcommittee on Retirement, Income and Employment*, 1975.

U.S. House Select Committee on Aging, U.S. House of Representatives, *Social Security Inequities against Women.* Washington, D.C., 1975.

U.S. Housing Acts of 1959 12 USC 1715 Z-1, as amended, Sections 202, 231 and 236.

U.S. Housing Act of 1978 P.L. 95-557; Sections 312 and 504.

U.S. Housing Act of 1978 P.L. 95-557; Congregate Housing Services Act; Title IV.

U.S. Housing and Community Development Act of 1974 42 USC 4501; esp. Section 8.

U.S. Senate Special Committee on Aging, *Hearings on the Adequacy of Federal Response to Housing Needs of Older Americans.* Washington, D.C., 1971-1976.

U.S. Senate Joint Economic Committee, *Hearings, Economic Problems of Women*, Washington, D.C., 1971.

U.S. Senate, Special Committee on Aging. *Developments in Aging: 1977.* Parts 1 and 2. Washington, D.C., 1978.

U.S. Senate, Special Committee on Aging. *Developments in Aging: 1978,* Parts 1 and 2. Washington, D.C., 1979.

U.S. Senate, Special Committee on Aging. "The Graying of Every Tenth American or Every Ninth American," by Herman B. Brotman, Consultant to Special Committee on Aging, *Developments in Aging*, 1978.

U.S. Senate, Special Committee on Aging. *Health Care for Older Americans: The Alternatives Issue, Hearings.* Washington, D.C., 16 May 1977.

U.S. Senate, Special Committee on Aging, *Home Health Services in the United States* Paper prepared by Brahna Trager. Washington, D.C., July 1973.

U.S. Senate, Special Committee on Aging. *New Perspectives in Health Care for Older Americans.* Report of Subcommittee on Health and Long-Term Care. Washington, D.C., January 1976.

U.S. Senate, Special Committee on Aging. "Protective Services for the Elderly." Paper prepared by John J. Regan and Georgia Springer. Washington, D.C., 1977.

U.S. Social Security Administration. "OASDI Digest." DHEW Publication (SSA) 74-11917. Washington, D.C.: U.S. Department of Health, Education and Welfare, 1974.

Van den Heuvel, W.J.A. "Older People and Their Health," *Some Notes on Health Measurement in Gerontology.* Nijmegan, Netherlands: Gerontologisch Centrum, 1974.

Wertheimer, Richard and Sheila Zedlewski, *Older American Reports*, 9 January 1980, p. 5.

White House Conference of 1961: "The Nation and Its Older People," World Health Organization, Regional Office for Europe, 1959; *The Public Health Aspects of the Aging of the Population*, Report of an advisory group, Oslo 28 July-2 August 1958. Copenhagen: World Health

Organization; *Technical Report Series 507.* Geneva: World Health
Organization; World Health Organization. *Planning and Organization
of Geriatric Services.* Technical Report, Series 548. Geneva: World
Health Organization.
White House Conference on Aging, "Toward a National Policy on Aging,"
Vol. 1, Background, Organization, Program. Washington, D.C., 1971.
Zimmer, Anna H., et al. *Incentives to Families Caring for Disabled Elderly:
Research and Demonstration Project to Strengthen the Natural Sup-
ports System.* Community Service Society of New York. Presented at
the 30th Annual Meeting of the Gerontological Society, San Francisco
Hilton, November 1977.

Index

About the Author

Louis Lowy (Ph.D., Harvard University) is professor and associate dean at Boston University School of Social Work and a member of the faculty of the Graduate School of Arts and Sciences. He is also a member and co-founder of the Boston University Gerontology Center. He served as its co-executive director from its founding in 1974 until 1977.

He has been chairperson of the Professional Advisory Committee of the Massachusetts Department of Elder Affairs since its inception in 1973 and was instrumental in designing the home-care programs for the state. He has been involved in gerontological social-work practice in a variety of social-service agencies and on policy-planning bodies in many parts of the country. He has acted as a consultant to community agencies here and abroad and has conducted a great number of educational programs and training activities throughout the United States and Canada as well as in West Germany, Switzerland, Norway, France, the Netherlands, and Israel. He has been an officer in the Gerontological Society and the National Association of Social Workers and has lectured extensively throughout this country and abroad. His latest publication, *Social Work with the Aging: The Challenge and Promise of the Later Years*, is one of a series of books and articles on gerontology, social work, and social-work education.